Are You Ready?

HOW TO PREPARE FOR AN
EARTHQUAKE

MAGGIE MOONEY

ARE YOU READY?

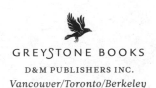

GREYSTONE BOOKS
D&M PUBLISHERS INC.
Vancouver/Toronto/Berkeley

Greystone Books
An imprint of D&M Publishers Inc.
2323 Quebec Street, Suite 201
Vancouver BC Canada V5T 4S7
www.greystonebooks.com

Cataloguing data available from Library and Archives Canada
ISBN 978-1-55365-850-4 (pbk.)
ISBN 978-1-55365-851-1 (ebook)

Editing by Barbara Tomlin
Illustrations by Mariko McCrae
Printed and bound in Canada by Friesens
Text printed on acid-free, 100% post-consumer paper
Distributed in the U.S. by Publishers Group West

We gratefully acknowledge the financial support of the Canada Council
for the Arts, the British Columbia Arts Council, the Province of British
Columbia through the Book Publishing Tax Credit, and the Government of
Canada through the Canada Book Fund for our publishing activities.

This book is dedicated to
the resilient people of Japan.

CONTENTS

ACKNOWLEDGEMENTS

THANKS TO Greystone Books for launching the project and in particular to Barbara Tomlin for her skilful editing. Barbara is a master of structure, and her respectful approach made the substantial reshaping of my writing much easier to take.

Thanks also to the book's reviewers: John Clague of the Centre for Natural Hazards Research at Simon Fraser University in Vancouver, B.C., and Teron Moore of Emergency Management British Columbia.

Gratitude also to my family and friends—my sister, Katherine, for making my work in Vancouver possible; Janet Lironi for some helpful coaching; the Saturday morning Artworks coffee circle for care and laughter; and especially to Michelle Benjamin—whose generosity is vaster than that of anyone I know—for her keen mind and sweet heart.

INTRODUCTION

A COUPLE of years ago I moved to an island off the coast of British Columbia. I was eager (and a little anxious) to experience one of the multiple power outages the island has each year. The previous owners left us a list of suggestions for preparing for an outage—how to tell when one was likely to happen (fierce winds, snow, heavy rain) and what to do before (fill the bathtub with water) and during (report the outage to the appropriate people). By the third outage I was a pro—I knew the signs that it was time to fill the tub with water and felt better knowing the flashlights were stored in various spots and the wood box was full so that I could cook on the wood stove if necessary. I realized that we were living in a culture of preparedness, and that being unprepared would not only look foolish to our new neighbours but would cause some fairly significant inconveniences. I also realized how much this culture of preparedness readied me for an event very likely to strike my west coast home: an earthquake.

Scientists who have spent their lives studying major geological events are convinced that a massive earthquake—the Big One—is imminent on the west coast of North America. And while the west coast is a seismically active area, earthquakes happen almost everywhere on our planet. The Earth is constantly moving in subtle and not-so-subtle ways. Recent events, including devastating earthquakes in Haiti, New Zealand, and Japan, have brought the threat of an earthquake to the forefront of our minds and raised our anxiety levels. But how many of us have actually responded by preparing ourselves for an earthquake happening close to where we live?

Earthquake expert John Clague watched the March 11, 2011, Japanese earthquake with keen interest. "We can't predict when the next one will occur," says the Simon Fraser University professor. "But," he continues, a seismic event is "inevitable... We *will* experience one, and... this earthquake [in Japan] is a perfect analog for what we would expect to see on our coast."

If a major earthquake knocked out your power, disrupted your water supply, and damaged your home, could you cope on your own for three days or more? A major earthquake would inevitably overwhelm local fire, police, and emergency services. Damage to transportation infrastructure and communication networks might mean that getting help would take hours or even days. Receiving requested assistance from neighbouring cities might also take days or even weeks. Clearly, help will be in short supply.

Getting Ready to Get Ready

Are You Ready? is actually two books in one: an introduction to the science of earthquakes and an emergency preparedness guide. After considering the awe-inspiring power of earthquakes, we look at the psychological and practical preparation needed to respond. Psychological preparation is particularly important because we need to know what holds us back from preparing before an earthquake strikes and what we are likely to think, feel, and do during and after a quake. Earthquake preparedness is about more than gathering supplies. Disaster research is a vast and lively field, and much has been discovered about how people—the prepared and the unprepared—respond. Understanding the psychological aspects of both anticipating and experiencing a life-threatening event will improve our ability to respond in an emergency.

The core of this book is a four-week readiness program that answers two important questions:

1. What are the minimum steps necessary to prepare for an earthquake?

2. How can busy people complete these most basic steps?

If you choose to follow this program, in week 1 you'll create an emergency communication plan and begin to put together the supplies you will need. In week 2 you'll identify and eliminate hazards from your home. In week 3 you'll practise the essential actions that should become second nature for you and your family during an earthquake. And in week 4 you'll look at safety issues involving your workplace and car. You'll also develop a plan for your pets if you need this.

In each week you'll use the checklists and forms provided here to simplify preparation. If you are a parent or you work with children, you will want to look at the "Tips for Children" sections included in most chapters. If at the end of four weeks you would like to do some advanced preparation, you can use the information included about earthquake-proofing your home.

Of course, you might be like my friend Jesse, who says, "Just give me the goods. I've got two kids under the age of six and I work full-time. I have no time to prepare!" Fine, I tell her, ignore the advanced preparation chapter and jump right past the science and psychology chapters to the four core readiness chapters. But the quick fix comes with a warning. The journey to the Land of Readiness is a tricky one. Many have travelled that route before and found themselves beached on the Isle of Procrastination—with drawers full of maps and checklists, a half-filled emergency kit, and little understanding of what to do when an earthquake hits. That's why this book includes a chapter on the psychology of preparing for and experiencing an earthquake. If you find yourself in a store, looking at bottles of water or first aid supplies, and the voice of that demon Anxiety whispers, "Oh! This is kind of scary. Why are you doing this anyway? Preparing is for dummies/losers/survivalist nuts," and then—overwhelmed by information, choices, and voices—you run out of steam, please do yourself and your wee ones a favour. Go back and read the earthquake psychology chapter, and then return to the readiness program when you're done. You'll thank me for it.

Taking Control

Injury—not death—is the main threat from an earthquake. Most injuries happen because people don't know what to do, and suffering can continue afterwards when people are not prepared to survive without help for the many hours or days required. Emergency preparedness experts recognize that both denial (believing a threat isn't real) and fatalism (assuming preparation won't make any difference) are common reactions that lead to taking unnecessary risks. The bottom line is that accidents—and disasters—happen. That's why we wear seat belts when we drive, and strap our children into safety seats. We're not acting out of fear, but out of love and a desire to do what is best for ourselves and our families. We never know what is going to happen next on this eventful planet. Instead of fearing what might happen, or burying our heads in the sand, we can take a healthier approach: we can prepare for the worst, then put it out of our minds and live for the best.

In my research I found numerous good sources of information. However, the material tended to fall into two camps: too detailed and complicated—the survivalist handbook that tells you how to perform surgery in the middle of a blizzard and asks you to devote yourself full-time to preparation; or too bare-bones—the how-to pamphlet that provides a list of emergency kit contents but no motivating explanations or background information.

Another problem with all the information available is that it overwhelms us with urgent demands to Do Something. What I offer here is a way to take control in a simple yet effective manner. By following the steps for each week you can prepare without exhausting yourself and terrifying your family.

Emergency planning and earthquake preparedness are being done all the time at an institutional level, and this is good. But—and it's a big *but*—experience and the actual history of disasters have repeatedly shown that the most effective first responses and best-sustained efforts have happened at the home and local community level.

What's the downside of preparing? You put time and effort into preparing and an earthquake doesn't happen in your lifetime. But you have candles ready if the power goes out, supplies in your car if you break down on the highway in winter, and an escape plan in place if your house is on fire and you need to get out quickly.

We are living on a moving, breathing, constantly expanding and contracting Earth. In choosing to prepare for an earthquake you will reduce a host of anxieties and be able to answer yes to that all-important question: Are you ready?

one

GEOLOGY 101
EARTHQUAKE BASICS

WHEN YOU think of an earthquake, what comes to mind? Scenes of people fleeing in panic? Cities washed out to sea? The Earth opening and swallowing buildings? Perhaps you think of movies you've seen or television programs about recent disasters in Japan, New Zealand, or Haiti. Perhaps you think further back, to the great San Francisco quake of 1906. For most of us, earthquakes are terrifying events. More than 3 million people were killed in quakes in the twentieth century alone. Yet for geologists, young children, poets, and of course for the Earth itself, an earthquake is not simply a disaster. It is a natural and awe-inspiring event. The tension between awesome and awful, between an eternity and today, between history and geology, has led some writers and scientists to use the term *geopoetry* to describe their understanding of earthquakes.

Geological Time

When we try to comprehend what actually happens in an earthquake, we enter geological time. This is a mind-twisting realm where vast floating landmasses propelled by inconceivable heat and pressure move in a slow, constant glide that takes place over thousands and millions of years.

Although we can't see the changes happening in human time, in geological time the Earth is constantly moving and evolving. We live on a giant flowing jigsaw puzzle, where the mountains, rivers, and the very land we live on and call home will likely not exist in the same form in the future. When I'm forced to confront this impermanence, I experience both wonder and fear—I get a kind of sick feeling, a bit like vertigo, in which the present sense of me and my existence speeds away into vast space.

The scale and enormity of these changes threaten our very security and make us feel like the fragile beings we are. Most of us would rather not think about the unsettling fact that our Earth is not only constantly changing but could destroy us in an instant. If we can for a moment accept the fact that the Earth is a moving dragon of sorts rather than a solid, stable mass, we can learn to ride this beast: to expect these movements and prepare to survive.

What Is an Earthquake?

The Earth—as ecologists always remind us—is alive, and an earthquake is the unfolding of a series of natural planetary events. An earthquake is merely a stretch or a shrug, one normal and expected movement among many. This is simply how the Earth behaves. Living things move. We are also living things who have decided to build our homes and other immense structures on the shoulders of this moving creature. Unfortunately, we often build right where earthquakes are most likely to happen—in the zones where stunning mountains and beautiful oceans meet.

In simplest terms, an earthquake is the sudden shaking of the ground caused by waves of energy moving through the Earth's crust. We imagine earthquakes as sudden events, yet an earthquake is actually a release of energy (geologists call it a strain) that has built up over decades or hundreds of years. Ultimately, it is the heat from the Earth's molten core that causes the movements that lead to earthquakes.

The Earth's Crust and Plate Tectonics
The surface of our planet is a thin crust of rock measuring a few kilometres thick in some places and about 100 kilometres (60 miles) thick in others, which protects us from the intense heat beneath—imagine a layer of ice atop a moving stream with water that grows progressively warmer the deeper you go. This crust and the layer beneath are always in motion. From a human perspective, the Earth's crust is a poor design. As geologist Robert Yeats humorously put it, "as an engineered structure, the Earth's crust is not up to code." Earthquakes happen because the crust—which itself is a multi-layered and complex structure—keeps failing.

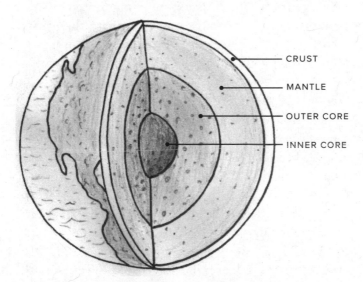

INSIDE THE EARTH. Seismic waves generated by the heat at our planet's core are felt on the surface as earthquakes.

According to the theory of plate tectonics, the Earth's crust comprises seven or eight (opinions differ) large plates—pieces of moving crust—and many smaller ones. They are separated by weak boundaries known as faults. Most of the time the motion of the plates, which are like overlapping puzzle pieces, is imperceptible to humans. For example, North America and Europe are slowly drifting apart at the rate of 5 centimetres (2 inches) per year.

Far below the plates is the Earth's core—an area the size of the moon with a solid inner sphere and a liquid outer layer. There, like the raging inferno in medieval portraits of hell, molten rock simmers away at temperatures around 5,500 degrees Celsius (10,000 degrees Fahrenheit). The heavy layers above (the mantle and crust) exert crushing pressure on the core and trap its heat, which in turn softens the surrounding rock and moves out towards the Earth's surface. The constant softening caused by heat radiating from the core causes rocks beneath the brittle crust to flow like superheated taffy. The motion leads to the buildup of energy within and between the plates floating above.

I thought of this energy recently as I watched a young tap dancer from New York; he never stopped moving and his legs never stopped shaking. Although he was entirely in control, he was always on the verge of losing his balance and falling. In the same way that this dancer shifted between stability and instability, the Earth's layers move constantly, always on the verge of slipping or exploding. And in the same way that the dancer interspersed his movements with loud syncopated taps or stamps, the Earth relieves the pressure that builds up within the crust with volcanic eruptions and earthquakes.

Ninety percent of earthquakes happen along the faults where stress builds up until something must give—either in a shift or a sudden break. Scientists have described these faults or boundaries along plates according to how the plates move against or around each other.

Faults along plates that slide horizontally past each other are called transform. The infamous San Andreas fault—the source of California's numerous earthquakes—is a transform fault. Plates also slide away from each other along what geologists call divergent boundaries. Africa's Great Rift Valley is an example of a divergent boundary. And plates can move beneath one another along what geologists call convergent boundaries The destruction of the Earth's crust happens most often, and most severely, at convergent boundaries, also called subduction zones—where one plate dives under (is subducted beneath) another. Subduction zones are the sites of the world's greatest earthquakes, with magnitudes of up to 9.5.

The Pacific Ring of Fire and Cascadia Subduction Zone
Earthquakes generally occur where two plates meet. One particularly intense area of tectonic activity is found along the edges of the giant Pacific plate, which lies beneath the Pacific Ocean. Activity in this so-called Ring of Fire causes earthquakes in Chile, Alaska, and Japan, and volcanic eruptions in the northwest United States, the Andes Mountains, and the Philippines. These events occur with the sudden slippage of faults separating adjacent plates. Earthquake activity in New Zealand and Indonesia, for example, is the result of friction between the Pacific plate and the Australian plate; activity along the San Andreas fault, which runs for roughly 1,300 kilometres (800 miles) through California, is the result of movement between the Pacific plate and the North American plate. Another volatile stretch of the Ring of Fire is just west and north of Haida Gwaii, off the British Columbia coast. There the Queen

Charlotte fault that lies between the Pacific and North American plates has produced a number of large earthquakes since record-keeping began and has the distinction of generating Canada's largest recorded earthquake—a magnitude 8.1 quake that struck in 1949.

The Cascadia subduction zone is part of the Ring of Fire and is located where the Juan de Fuca plate and some smaller plates are being driven eastward beneath the North American plate. This zone runs for more than 1,100 kilometres (680 miles), from the north of Vancouver Island to the south just off Cape Mendocino in California. There it intersects the San Andreas fault and the Mendocino fault zone.

When I was growing up in Vancouver in the 1970s, earthquakes weren't a particular cause for concern. I remember fire drills at school but never earthquake drills. I do remember experiencing some shaking, but it was just something that happened once in a while, and it was kind of fun. Real earthquakes happened in the movies or in South America or Japan.

Until the early 1980s, scientists were not aware that a major subduction earthquake might occur in the Pacific Northwest. Scientists interpreted the absence of large non-crustal earthquakes in the area as evidence that this was a smooth transition zone where plates glided effortlessly under one another, and they assumed there was little threat.

More recently, though—1987 was the start of a shift in thinking—scientists moved from believing there was no threat to being certain that there is a major threat. Geologists discovered that in fact the plates are not moving smoothly; rather, they are stuck. The plates have not been producing earthquakes because they are—for now—locked in place. As we know, the Earth is always moving, and when it can't move pressure or strain builds up. This pressure continues to build and must eventually be released.

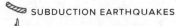
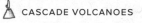

⊙ DEEP EARTHQUAKES
• SHALLOW EARTHQUAKES
〰 SUBDUCTION EARTHQUAKES
△ CASCADE VOLCANOES

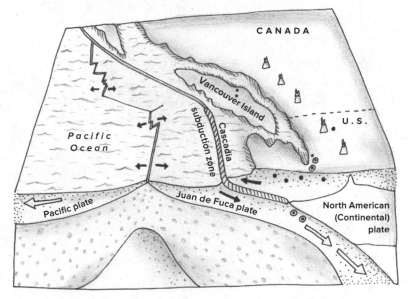

CASCADIA SUBDUCTION ZONE. As the large North American plate moves southwest, the small Juan de Fuca plate slides east and underneath (subducts) the North American plate.

And when the pressure of all those years is released—remember we're talking geological time here—the Big One will be upon us. The Cascadia subduction zone has the potential to produce very large megathrust earthquakes. Subduction zone earthquakes are the largest in the world, and can exceed magnitude 9.0. The 2011 Japan earthquake was a subduction zone event.

The Cascadia subduction zone, which includes the entire Lower Mainland of British Columbia, Seattle, Washington, and Portland, Oregon, is one of the most seismically active regions in the world. Small earthquakes occur almost daily, and more than one hundred earthquakes with a magnitude of 5.0 or greater (most offshore) have occurred in the past seventy years. Everyone in this area must be prepared for more earthquakes.

Do We Know When an Earthquake Will Happen?

Can scientists predict earthquakes? If you mean can they tell us exactly where and when an earthquake will happen, and what the magnitude of such a quake will be, then the answer is no—they can't predict.

However, they are increasingly able to forecast *where* an earthquake is likely to occur in a region. We slip back into geological time here, and focus on probability. If a fault has not experienced movement in millions of years then the probability of movement anytime soon is low. But some faults have experienced movement more recently, over the last two thousand years, for example, so that a pattern emerges and higher-probability forecasts can be made.

So what are scientists saying about the likelihood of a major earthquake in the Pacific Northwest? Some forecast a magnitude 8.0 quake will happen on just part of the fault—the southern portion, say from Northern California to mid-Oregon. Others predict it will be a massive magnitude 9.0 or higher event along the entire length of the fault up to northern Vancouver Island. The majority of scientists favour the magnitude 9.0 option.

Seismologists studying the region base their forecast on an analysis of previous subduction earthquakes that have occurred. Geologists tell us that twenty great subduction earthquakes have occurred in the Pacific Northwest in the past ten thousand years—one every five hundred years, on average. The last one, which had a magnitude greater than 9.0, occurred in 1700. Through studying the way past earthquakes cluster, scientists have developed a probability curve that shows a fifty percent chance of a megathrust earthquake occurring here in the next two hundred years, and a thirty percent chance of such an earthquake occurring within the next fifty years. Of course, this is all just probability. Such a quake might also happen tomorrow.

How Are Earthquakes Measured?

Earthquakes are recorded by an instrument called a seismometer (earlier versions are known as seismographs) that measures the seismic waves caused by the sudden breaking of rock within the Earth. Seismic waves can take two forms: body waves, which move through the solid Earth, and surface waves, which, as the name suggests, travel across the surface of the Earth. The seismometer measures two kinds of body waves—P-waves (P for primary—these are the first waves sent out by an earthquake) and S-waves (S for secondary). Think of P-waves as push-pull waves and S-waves as shear or side-to-side waves.

Seismometers are positioned in locations throughout a known earthquake territory. The seismometer's base is set firmly in the ground, while a heavy weight hangs free within the instrument. When the ground shakes, the base of the seismograph also shakes, but the hanging weight does not; instead, the spring or string that it hangs from absorbs the movement. The instrument then records the difference in position between the moving weight and the motionless base. These recordings of movement are called seismograms, and most are now recorded digitally.

The magnitude or size of an earthquake depends on the amount of movement along a fault and the area over which the movement occurs. Scientists cannot easily measure this movement since faults can be many kilometres deep beneath the Earth's surface. Instead, they use the seismo-grams made at the surface of the Earth to determine the size of an earthquake. Weak ground shaking over a small area means a small earthquake, and strong, long-duration shaking over a large area means a large earthquake.

The destructive power of an earthquake depends on the depth of its source, also called the focus. For the most common quakes, known as shallow events, the focus is less than 10 kilometres (6 miles) below the surface. These can be powerful and deadly quakes if they occur near populated areas. The Haiti earthquake in 2010 and the Christchurch, New Zealand, earthquake in 2011 are examples. In contrast, deep-focus earthquakes originate many kilometres below the surface and cause less damage. Earthquakes also occur beneath the ocean, where they can trigger enormous waves called tsunamis that travel great distances at extraordinary speeds and reach great heights when they run ashore. Whether quakes occur beneath ocean or land, the spot on the Earth's surface directly above the focus is called the epicentre.

The Modified Mercalli Scale

The Mercalli scale was invented by Italian volcanologist Giuseppe Mercalli in 1902 and later modified by German, English, and American scientists. This scale uses the observations of the people who experienced the earthquake to estimate its intensity.

The Modified Mercalli scale measures how people feel and react to the shaking of an earthquake and is based on a series of key responses, such as people awakening, furniture moving, and damage occurring to structures. It is a relative scale because people experience different amounts of shaking in different places. The Modified Mercalli scale isn't considered as scientific as the Richter or Moment

Magnitude scale since it is based on subjective observation rather than scientific measurement. As well, the amount of damage caused by the earthquake may not accurately reflect how strong it was.

The Richter Scale

The scale familiar to most of us is the Richter scale, invented by American seismologist Charles Richter in 1934. Richter's intention was to measure the range of medium-sized earthquakes in southern California. For this he needed a more scientific scale, one based on mathematical measurements rather than on the subjective observations of the Modified Mercalli. The Richter scale measures an earthquake's magnitude—the intensity of the shaking—on a seismograph or seismometer. It is actually a measurement of the height (amplitude) of the waves produced by the earthquake.

Richter magnitudes are based on a logarithmic scale (base 10). This means that for each whole number you move up on the Richter scale, the amplitude of the motion recorded by a seismograph goes up ten times. In other words, a magnitude 5.0 earthquake expresses ten times the level of ground shaking as a magnitude 4.0 earthquake. The Richter scale works well on small and medium earthquakes but becomes unreliable in large earthquakes. However, because it can be calculated quickly—something appreciated by the media   you will still often hear a Richter scale number reported.

The Moment Magnitude Scale

Contemporary seismologists use the Moment Magnitude scale to measure earthquakes. Two earthquakes in the twentieth century—the 1960 Chile earthquake and 1964 Alaska earthquake—were both too large to measure accurately using the Richter scale. In response, seismologists

Thomas C. Hanks and Hiroo Kanamori developed the Moment Magnitude scale in the 1970s. This more complex and more consistent scale measures the amount of energy released during an earthquake by considering the length of the fault that ruptures, the zone of aftershocks, and the physical changes—such as surface slip—that occur. The way the Richter and Moment Magnitude scales differ can be seen by referring to the 1964 Alaska earthquake. With a fault rupture area the size of Iowa, this quake measured 9.2 on the Moment Magnitude scale but only 8.5 on the Richter scale. Although seismologists no longer use the Richter scale for measuring large earthquakes, the public and the media have both been slow to let go of the more familiar Richter.

EARTHQUAKE INTENSITY AND MAGNITUDE

Modified Mercalli Intensity	Equivalent Richter Magnitude	Witness Observations
I	1.0 to 2.0	Moderate, no damage. Felt by very few people; barely noticeable.
II	2.0 to 3.0	Moderate, no damage. Felt by a few people, especially on upper floors.
III	3.0 to 4.0	Moderate, no damage. Noticeable indoors, especially on upper floors, but may not be recognized as an earthquake.
IV	4.0	Moderate, no damage. Felt by many indoors, few outdoors. May feel like a heavy truck passing by.
V	4.0 to 5.0	Rather strong. Felt by almost everyone, some people awakened. Damage negligible. Small, unstable objects displaced or upset. Some dishes and glassware broken.

Modified Mercalli Intensity	Equivalent Richter Magnitude	Witness Observations
VI	5.0 to 6.0	Strong. Felt by everyone. Difficult to stand. Some heavy furniture moved. Some plaster falls. Chimneys may be slightly damaged.
VII	6.0	Very Strong. Slight to moderate damage in well-built, ordinary structures. Considerable damage to poorly built structures. Some walls may fall.
VIII	6.0 to 7.0	Destructive. Little damage in specially built structures; considerable damage to ordinary buildings; severe damage to poorly built structures. Some walls collapse.
IX	7.0	Ruinous. Considerable damage to specially built structures. Buildings shifted off foundations. Ground cracked noticeably. Landslides.
X	7.0 to 8.0	Disastrous. Most masonry and frame structures and their foundations destroyed. Ground badly cracked. Landslides. Wholesale destruction.
XI	8.0	Very Disastrous. Total damage. Few or no structures standing. Bridges destroyed. Wide cracks in ground. Waves seen on ground.
XII	8.0 or greater	Catastrophic. Total damage. Waves seen on ground. Objects thrown up into air.

EARTHQUAKE FREQUENCY BY MAGNITUDE		
Magnitude	Effects	Estimated Number of Earthquakes Each Year
2.5 or less	Usually not felt, but can be recorded by seismograph.	900,000
2.5 to 5.4	Often felt, but only causes minor damage.	30,000
5.5 to 6.0	May cause slight damage to buildings and other structures.	500
6.1 to 6.9	May cause a lot of damage in very populated areas.	100
7.0 to 7.9	Major earthquake. Causes serious damage.	20
8.0 or greater	Great earthquake. Can totally destroy communities near the epicentre.	One every 5 to 10 years

How Do We Know Where the Earthquake Happened?

Seismograms can be used to identify the location as well as the size of an earthquake. The principle is similar to the one that helps us identify the centre of a thunderstorm. During a storm we see the lightning first and hear the thunder later because light travels faster than sound. The closer we are to the lightning at the centre of the storm, the sooner we hear the boom of the accompanying thunder. The farther we are from the storm's centre, the longer the gap between the lightning and the thunder. During an earthquake, P-waves are like the lightning and S-waves are like the thunder. The P-waves travel faster and arrive first at the seismometer. The S-waves follow. If we are close to the earthquake, the

P-waves and S-waves will come one right after the other, but if we are far away, there will be more time between the two. By examining the amount of time between the two kinds of waves as recorded on a seismogram, scientists can tell how far away the earthquake was from the seismometer.

Seismologists can also determine where the earthquake occurred in relation to the seismometer by drawing concentric circles on a map around affected seismology stations. The point where those circles intersect is the epicentre.

EARTHQUAKE LIGHTS

For millennia, observers have described startling flashes and sheets of radiance at the time of an earthquake. Once thought to be hallucinations or the stuff of myth, earthquake lights are now acknowledged to be true phenomena, although the cause of these displays has not been determined.

Earthquake lights are generally blue and white gaseous plasmas or luminous bands that appear before, during, and after seismic activity. At times, especially at night, they can resemble the aurora borealis. They can also take the form of fiery floating balls or flames shooting skyward. Some researchers suggest that earthquake lights result from flammable gases released from natural gas pockets below the Earth's surface, while others theorize that the electrical characteristics of the rocks themselves transform under the severe seismic stress and generate charges, which ionize the gases and produce glowing lights.

---

two

EARTHQUAKE PSYCHOLOGY

WE KNOW that we should prepare for an earthquake, especially if we live on the west coast of North America, yet few of us have done more than take a few first steps. We've vowed to get prepared and have even gone so far as to make a list or put away a bottle of water or a few tins of emergency food. For most of us, however—including me before this writing project provided the motivation I needed—something happens and we stop preparing.

When I began to work on this book, I assumed it was pure busyness that stopped me and my friends and neighbours from preparing. We are busy people living in a busy time. We are constantly distracted—the report is due tomorrow, the clutter in the basement needs sorting, or the kids need a ride to soccer practice. We simply don't have time. But there is more than busyness involved.

Earthquakes present a problem for the human mind. These awe-inspiring events happen daily and by the thousands each year on our planet. When they are large they bring untold misery and years of reconstruction for communities. The problem is that although we know the threat is real and through the news we can often witness the terrible effects, the uncertainty and unpredictability of earthquakes provoke feelings of unreality and distance. The enormous power of an earthquake challenges our imaginations.

What We Do in an Earthquake

The rich field of inquiry known as disaster research has drawn on sociological and psychological investigations, including studies of brain function, to give us a better picture of how humans behave during a catastrophic situation. The results indicate few of us act as we assume we will and strongly support the need to prepare for the overwhelming effects of a natural disaster.

What we've learned from research on effective responses to disasters is now used when training the first-responders we rely upon to keep their heads during a crisis—police officers, fire fighters, paramedics, and members of the military. These and other rescue personnel use the seven *P*'s mnemonic—"Proper planning and preparation prevents piss-poor performance"—and rehearse repeatedly during real-time disaster simulations. This allows them to respond from body or muscle memory when under extreme stress. While we civilians don't necessarily need the skills and instincts of a first-responder, we can still benefit from some of the techniques emergency professionals use to cope in the midst of a crisis. By anticipating and rehearsing for situations that frighten and threaten us, we will feel less scared and will respond better during a disaster.

Risk Perception

If we are aware that we live in an earthquake zone and we are also aware that preparing for a disaster can greatly

reduce the scale of damage and loss, then we'll prepare. Right? Not necessarily. Awareness is important, but
when it comes to preparation there is a surprisingly poor
relationship between awareness and action. This is why
some people remain in their homes even as they watch
flood waters rise around them or hurricane force winds
rip the siding off their houses. Research indicates that
regardless of our knowledge and experience, we tend to
under-perceive the risk of disaster striking us.

A leading disaster expert in the U.S., Dennis Mileti, was
heartbroken by Hurricane Katrina. He knew that the suffering could have been avoided. "How many citizens must
die? How many people do you need to see pounding through
their roofs?" he asked. "We know exactly—*exactly*—where
the major disasters will occur...But individuals under-
perceive risk."

This human tendency to under-perceive risk is illus-
trated by the small village of Máncora on the north coast
of Peru, where my family volunteered a couple of years ago.
In Máncora, buildings range from flimsy shacks built on or
below desert hillsides to large expensive hotels built right
on the beach. Every ten years, major flooding related to an
El Niño occurs and reshapes the coastline. Inevitably, the
hotels are damaged, the town is flooded, and the hillside
shacks are destroyed. And inevitably, everything is rebuilt
in the same precarious locations.

What's operating here is the human tendency to assess
risk based on our likes and dislikes rather than by weighing the true advantages and disadvantages. In other words,
we perceive and judge by our preferences rather than by
the facts. For example, if I asked the villagers in Máncora to
name the positive and negative aspects of life in their village, they would glowingly report on the beaches, the sun,

and the tasty ceviche. Very few, if any, would mention the cyclical flooding and landslides that shift their coastline and destroy their buildings when an El Niño arrives.

How this applies to earthquakes is easy to see. We do not look clearly at the risks involved in living where we do. Few residents of Vancouver or Seattle asked about the benefits and risks of living where they do would include earthquakes as a cost of living in Lotus Land.

Optimistic Bias and Denial

At the same time we under-perceive risk, we tend to overestimate how well we will function during a disaster. Many of us have a vague sense that we will be fine in the event of an earthquake. We assume that somehow we will instinctively or intuitively know what to do to survive. This, of course, is foolish. Optimism is a wonderful and necessary trait, but the active looking away from risk—denial—reduces our ability to respond effectively. If we optimistically believe that our common sense will tell us how to respond in the moment of an earthquake, we are far more likely to act on our first "common sense" impulse and run outside when a building starts to shake—the most natural and often the worst thing you can do.

Making optimistic assumptions and under-perceiving risk puts us in a fantasy world where we can convince ourselves that (1) an earthquake isn't really going to happen and (2) we can deal with it if it does. This can only lead to trouble. Just ask those overly optimistic risk-takers who go hiking or skiing in the back country every year without being prepared, assuming they will be rescued if they run into difficulties. Or ask your optimistic friend who was recently diagnosed with lung disease after years of cigarette smoking that she claimed was having no ill effects.

Optimism is healthy—we don't want to become overly preoccupied with risk. But unthinking optimism is a dangerous thing.

The Experience of an Earthquake

There's no single experience of an earthquake, but many people who have survived a major quake describe a similar set of sensations and reactions. Here's what journalist Michael Ventura experienced during the 1994 Northridge earthquake in Los Angeles:

Without warning in the dark there was the shaking, everything shuddering, shivering, the bed, the walls. There was the shock of being suddenly and absolutely awake, as awake as it is possible to be, with no residue of sleep... In the moment, it was one's animal body in pure wakefulness.

In the same instant there was the sense of trying to see what we could not see in a dark room, a dark world, a world of trembling shadows. And it was not only the world that trembled, it was us—our bodies were both being shaken by the quake and shaking within, a double onslaught. Then to bolt from bed naked, stand in the doorway, shout to each other, we had to shout for there was a great sound. We were shaking and the walls were shaking, so this sound seemed to come as much from within as without. It was as though we were shouting over ourselves, through ourselves. Shouting each other's names...

Then came the surge. Walls that had been shaking now were jolting, the floor was bouncing, it was hard to stand up and everything was crashing. There was the sound of many things breaking, the sound of the walls as they strained, and beyond all this another sound, unthinkable, indescribable. It was the sound of the quake itself, a sound from deep in the Earth.

Then the building stopped shaking but we didn't. This was also terribly strange, fumbling with our clothes in the dark amid broken glass, as though we'd forgotten how to get dressed.

From somewhere not far off there was a huge explosion. It sounded like (and turned out to be) a house falling down. Then we waited, outside, in the chill of early morning. But my body was colder than the dawn chill could account for—I was stone-cold with shock.

We sat in the car, the heater going full blast, but I couldn't get warm. I could function, but I couldn't stop myself from freezing. And while we waited, it quaked some more. They call them "aftershocks," but it feels like, and is, more quakes. That morning they were very strong, rocking the car back and forth as though it were held in some great hand and being toyed with.

Ventura's fascinating and terrifying account shows what an overwhelming threat an earthquake poses for the human psyche. The earth is shaking, walls and floors are straining, objects are crashing, and the sounds are deafening and disorienting. Without having prepared ourselves through practice we may not do the right things to protect ourselves and our loved ones.

The Brain in an Earthquake

Brain research done over the last two decades has given us insight into how people commonly respond to the stress of a major crisis such as an earthquake. To begin with, the shaking sets off an immediate and complicated physiological response. The oldest part of our brain—the amygdala, located in the medial temporal lobe and responsible for our emotional reactions—takes over. It shoots hormones (cortisol and other stress hormones) into our brain to prepare us for the classic fight, flight, or freeze response. This instinctive response has worked well for humans throughout our evolution. When confronted by a wild animal or a knife-wielding human, the rest of our brain shuts down to allow us to focus all energy and attention on the threat. This happens automatically, often before we become fully aware of the threat.

In the case of an earthquake, unless we've practised beforehand and actually trained ourselves to respond appropriately while in a relaxed state, we are in danger of fleeing in panic—this is the irresistible urge to run outside that virtually everyone feels when the ground-shifting movement of an earthquake begins. We are also in danger of being overcome by fear and dread. The stress hormones are fed back to the amygdala, making the fear even stronger, and we can get locked into a cycle of increasing and paralyzing terror. Our sense of time slows down and our thinking becomes more and more difficult. This can ultimately lead to an extremely dangerous trance-like state where we freeze and do nothing.

Understanding Anxiety and Fatalism

The responses revealed by brain research and described by disaster survivors—the surge of adrenaline, the fluctuating body temperature, the overwhelming sense of fear and dread—are extreme expressions of anxiety. A less intense but equally dangerous kind of anxiety is inspired by thinking about an unpredictable and potentially devastating natural disaster. This kind of anxiety can lead eventually to denial or a fatalistic acceptance of danger.

Eric Holdeman, former director of emergency management for Seattle's King County, provides a succinct model of how fatalism develops. He says we cope with anxiety about disasters by telling ourselves:

1. A disaster won't happen (denial).

2. If it does happen, it won't happen to me (optimistic bias).

3. If it does happen to me, it won't be that bad (denial and optimistic bias).

4. If it happens to me and it's bad, there's nothing I can do to stop it anyway (fatalism).

Fatalism is especially dangerous because it translates into inaction. If you maintain the belief there's nothing you can do, you will not take steps to do what is actually within your control. Even in situations where many have died, many more have survived because they were prepared and they took the right actions.

Fostering Resilience

As well as accepting the fact that bad things happen and we should prepare for them, we need to develop greater psychological resilience—the ability to spring back from and adapt to hardships. When it comes to surviving an earthquake, resilience is key. We all have different personalities and temperaments and each of us has developed in family and community contexts that vary regarding the cultivation of resilience. However, we can actively build resilience in the same way we build competence in any skill—through observing models of resilience and through practice.

Japan: A Model of Resilience

If you aren't sure what resilience looks like, simply consider the way Japan responded to a triple disaster in March 2011—megathrust earthquake, tsunami, and nuclear power plant crisis. During the initial reporting of these events, I felt frustration along with shock and heartbreak. Not only was the suffering difficult to witness, but many media reports presented a one-sided story of hopelessness and chaos. This kind of reporting suggests there is little point in preparing for an earthquake because the consequences are outside our control. In reality, the situation would have been far, far worse if the Japanese people had not been prepared. Thousands—perhaps hundreds of thousands—of lives were saved because people knew what to do. Children followed instructions to take cover, buildings didn't collapse because they had been properly constructed, and although the magnitude 9.0 quake (the fourth largest in recorded history) outstripped even Japanese expectations, an early warning system that is the most advanced in the world quickly alerted millions to the possibility of tsunamis—including my daughter, who was on the west coast of Vancouver Island—a tsunami hazard zone—that morning.

Japan has lived for centuries with both natural and human-made calamities: volcanic eruptions, typhoons, floods, earthquakes, tsunamis, war, and the atomic bombing of Hiroshima and Nagasaki. No matter the level of devastation, the Japanese have demonstrated again and again an unmatched ability to bounce back and rebuild their society. Cultural identity is a complex subject, but for our purposes it is useful to highlight the realistic perception of risk held by the Japanese and the culture of preparedness this has inspired. The Japanese accept the fact that they live on a volatile chain of islands, and they have a history of improving survival rates with advanced building codes and preparation rituals in families and communities. On September 1 each year, hundreds of thousands of people participate in Disaster Preparedness Day, which includes elaborate rehearsals for emergencies and commemorations for those lost in past disasters.

The focus on planning and the cultivation of resilience in Japan are both aspects of a cultural concept called *gambaru*—a word often translated as "never give up." Shortly after the March 2011 earthquake we saw *gambaru* in action as Twitter messages calling for persistence and tenacity in the face of terrible circumstances flew from one end of the country to the other.

Ways to Become More Resilient
To be psychologically prepared when disaster strikes, you can follow the Japanese example and become more resilient.

> **Watch your attitude.** Those who do best after disasters believe they have some level of control, whatever the circumstances, and thus never give up. They also look for what they can learn, just as the Japanese continue to learn more from each calamity. You can't control life-threatening events, but you can change how you interpret and respond to them. Practise during lesser crises by telling yourself over and over that there is always something you can do, looking for what you can control as well as what you can learn from whatever difficulty you're dealing with.

> **Get to know your neighbours.** People with strong support systems do well in adversity. Emergency services may not reach you for hours or days after a quake, so get to know your neighbours and co-workers, the most important people next to your immediate family during the aftermath of a disaster.

> **Plan and take decisive actions.** Rather than denying you live where disaster might strike (that is, anywhere), take decisive steps to prepare. The more prepared you are, the more control you will have. The more control you have, the better you will perform during an earthquake or other emergency. Your responsibility is to be prepared, to have a clear plan, and to have on hand the supplies you'll need to survive until help arrives.

> **Be goal directed.** Move step by step towards a realistic goal and reward yourself for each small accomplishment. This will help develop self-confidence in your abilities.

> **Take care of yourself.** Those who do best after disasters are usually physically fit. Having to survive outdoors in mid-winter or evacuate on foot carrying supplies are both very real possibilities. Try to improve your level of fitness and maintain or attain a healthy body weight. Also, find ways to enjoy life and experience calm and connection, perhaps through meditation and spiritual or creative practices.

> **Keep things in perspective.** I've always been amazed by the ability of Japanese people to keep a long term perspective on what has happened to them. After each crisis they have immediately turned their attention to the future and how they will rebuild their shattered world. Keep them in mind when difficult events happen in your life and avoid blowing the event out of proportion.

> **Breathe.** Learn to calm yourself with the breathing techniques described on pages 42 and 43.

Situational Awareness
In the event of a disaster, you will have a better chance of survival if you are fully aware of whatever situation you are in at the time. This "situational awareness" is simply

knowing what's going on around you so that you can determine the best response and act without surprise. For instance, once or twice a month I commute from my home on a small island off the coast of British Columbia to the city of Vancouver. Often this has me using many kinds of transport, including ferry, taxi, float plane, subway, and bus, and walking through urban, suburban, and rural settings. In an effort to develop my situational awareness, I scan buildings for exits, review maps, and actually listen when the float plane pilot describes the location of emergency exits. I also think about where I would seek shelter if the ground started to shake and I had to do the most important thing:

- Drop to my hands and knees (preferably underneath a sturdy table or desk—see page 74).

- Cover my head and neck with my arms.

- Hold on to the most secure object available.

Reacting appropriately under stress is challenging for all of us, as the experience of a geologist and author of several books on earthquakes demonstrates. Robert Yeats was sitting in a hotel bar in Mexico City when he noticed the chandelier start to sway. At first he thought he was imagining things. Then the waves struck. "Glasses and bottles toppled from the bar, chairs scraped back, and people began to yell in Spanish. The entire building began to rumble, like the noise of a train. *Earthquake,* I thought."

The knowledgeable earthquake specialist knew what was happening, yet the next moment—against all his training—he found himself running outside. "I knew that it was the wrong thing to do, but rational behavior fled with the strong shaking. Fortunately, we were not bombarded by masonry or plate glass."

Yeats's story illustrates the need to train yourself to react appropriately for the time when disaster strikes. Running is almost always the wrong thing to do. The right thing is to drop, cover, and hold on—something you should practise at home, at work, and wherever else you spend time. Remember that you will not have time to stop and think. When an earthquake happens you want muscle memory to take over.

Creating a Culture of Preparedness

The principles and practices of earthquake preparedness in this book are part of a larger shift in public thinking. It is becoming far more common for governments and organizations to focus on preventing harm in the first place—to be proactive rather than reactive about illness and injury. We have education campaigns that remind us about the effects of smoking, the need for a nutritious diet, and the importance of seat belts and smoke detectors. This is largely because we've learned that preventing harm is more effective than treating ills after the fact. And we've learned that along with public health campaigns and fire drills, we need earthquake drills.

The first Great Southern California ShakeOut event was held in 2008. During that ShakeOut and subsequent ones, participants practised doing what they should during a quake—at a designated time millions found their way under tables and desks and waited until the "shaking" stopped. Dr. Lucy Jones, a seismologist with the U.S. Geological Survey and one of the scientists behind the ShakeOut program, envisions a time when children will come home from school and say, "We had an earthquake drill at school today," and a parent will respond, "I had one at work today too," and a discussion on earthquakes and preparation plans involving the whole family will follow. Jones says, "sociologists tell us that when we talk about [earthquakes] with people we care about, it becomes an issue we're really willing to work on."

After the first British Columbia ShakeOut in 2011, I spoke to a number of people about their experience. A common response was that the exercise was a bit disappointing—a letdown after a big buildup. One friend said, "We got under our desks and held on, and that was it. I expected someone to tell us what to do, to lead us through an emergency." However, as we talked more about his "disappointing" experience, my friend realized that he and everyone else who participated in ShakeOut had actually done the most important thing they could—drop, cover, and hold on— during a time when adrenaline wasn't pumping through their veins. When an earthquake actually happens, instead of running screaming into the streets, my friend will remember what he needs to do and he'll have a better chance of staying safe. His muscle memory will take over. What happens during an earthquake isn't about following instructions because there won't be a big voice telling us what to do—only our own well-prepared inner voice.

It's perfectly rational to be fearful and anxious about earthquakes—they involve huge forces and it's natural to feel powerless when faced with the prospect of one. However, we are not powerless and the more we prepare, the more our ability to cope and survive increases. This applies especially when it comes to our children.

Preparing Children

For most parents and grandparents, children provide the strongest motivation to get ready for an earthquake. We may be inclined to put any risk to ourselves out of mind, but this is not the case when it comes to our children. We are both protectors of our children and models for them.

We should have two goals in mind as we prepare children for an earthquake. The first and most obvious is to ensure they know what to expect and do during and after an earthquake. The second goal is to make preparedness part of family habits and traditions. Educate children early so that they are emotionally, intellectually, and physically prepared. Even young children can learn to dial 9-1-1 and participate in making plans and assembling supplies. When you live in an earthquake zone or anywhere else emergencies can occur, preparing your children is not an extreme or paranoid response.

Talk about Earthquakes
Children can develop strange ideas about what causes earthquakes, similar to the misconceptions around sex they may pick up in the schoolyard. How they misunderstand earthquakes can include viewing them as caused by a supernatural force or some bad human behaviour, especially their own.

When I first mentioned to friends that I was writing a book about emergency preparedness, stories of childhood anxieties flowed forth. One friend told me she used to lie awake night after night worrying about fire and whether she should leave her bedroom door open or closed. As a little girl, my friend was tormented by contradictory advice: she had heard that she should close the door and put a towel underneath to keep out smoke, but she also knew she was supposed to get out fast in the case of fire, and how could she do that if the door was closed?

This sparked a memory of my own recurring childhood fear connected with the storm cellar scene in *The Wizard of Oz*. Somehow I had the strange notion that I would have to answer a skill-testing question to be admitted to an emergency shelter like the one used by Dorothy's family—and I was terrified that I wouldn't know the answer. My anxiety was not surprising given that when I grew up the Cuban Missile Crisis had led people to build bomb shelters in their backyards. But children in any era can harbour misunderstandings and fears. It is important to talk about possible emergency events like earthquakes regularly so that you know about your child's misconceptions and anxieties as they arise. Talking about scary things takes away their power.

Engage the Imagination

When preparing for possible emergencies, start by engaging your child's imagination. Reading legends about earthquakes from cultures around the world (see pages 44–45) can be a good way to introduce young children to the subject. You might also read aloud the following story, which is thought to have originated with the Gabrielino Indians whose ancestral home is in the San Gabriel Valley of southern California.

Once, a long time ago, before there was land or people and the world was made only of water, Great Spirit looked down from above. He wanted to create a beautiful land but didn't know where to start. As he looked out over the expanse of water, he spotted a turtle. This was a giant turtle—as big as an enormous island—and so Great Spirit thought he might try to make the beautiful land on the turtle's back.

But even though this was a huge turtle, Great Spirit wanted to make a very large land, so he called to the giant turtle to gather his six brothers. The giant turtle swam great distances to find his brothers. On the first day he found one of his brothers, and by the end of the second day he had found another. In all, it took six days to find all six brothers.

When Great Spirit saw that the seven turtles had gathered, he called to them, "Turtles! You must help me to create a beautiful land." And Great Spirit directed the giant turtles to take their places in the expanse of water. Head to tail, north to south, side by side, east to west, Great Spirit organized the giant turtles.

The giant turtles stayed very still as Great Spirit placed a layer of straw on their backs. On top of the straw he added a layer of rich soil. He pulled thick white clouds from the sky and used them to form majestic mountains. Then Great Spirit created trees and plants, lakes and rivers. When he finished, he looked down at the beautiful land and was pleased. He said, "It is a great honour to carry this land on your backs and so from this day on you must not move."

But trouble was ahead. The giant turtles had been still for too long, and their legs were growing restless. They needed to stretch and wiggle, and they became irritated with one another. "I want to swim towards the east," said one. "I want to move west," said another, "towards the setting sun."

The turtles began to argue with one another and could not agree about which direction they should travel. One day, four of the turtle brothers began to swim to the east while the other three swam to the west. The beautiful land created by Great Spirit started to shake. It cracked with a loud noise! But the giant turtles had to stop moving because the land on their backs was too heavy. They had only been able to swim a small distance from each other, and so the shaking stopped after just a moment.

When the turtle brothers realized that they could not swim away, they stopped arguing and settled down into their places. Every once in a while, though, the turtles who hold up the land of California stretch and wiggle and argue again. Each time they do, the Earth shakes for a few moments.

Make Preparation Age-Appropriate

Once you have introduced the subject, find out what your children already know about earthquakes and then help them learn more. Visit your local library to borrow books about earthquake science and geology. Older kids might enjoy science experiments that simulate the effects of an earthquake or tsunami. One example I've seen demonstrates liquefaction by bouncing a wheelbarrow of mud down the street. The mud turns to liquid with the shaking and then firms up when the wheelbarrow comes to rest.

Emphasize the naturalness of such processes and encourage children to be impressed by the awe-inspiring energy coming from the Earth's core. Remember to be impressed yourself and keep your fears in check. When your child is fearful and asks, "What will happen to me when an earthquake comes?" you need to manage your own anxiety and use such questions as an opportunity to discuss emergency plans.

Whatever books you read and whatever activities you undertake, emphasize being in control—an earthquake or other natural disaster may be scary, but together you can prepare. As you reassure your children of any age that they will be looked after, you can also imbue "getting ready" with a sense of adventure. For example, as you complete the readiness program described in the chapters that follow, you might introduce each week's tasks in terms of a family activity:

- Week 1: Let's make a staying-in-touch plan.

- Week 2: Let's hunt for earthquake hazards in the living room.

- Week 3: Let's practise "drop, cover, and hold on" in the kitchen.

- Week 4: Let's make an emergency plan for Fido.

With small children, don't get too hung up on emergency plan details or scientific explanations. Simply address anxieties that arise by correcting misconceptions and providing explanations that they can understand. This will be an ongoing conversation so don't feel you have to pile on the facts. Children are concrete thinkers; they will turn the abstractions you offer, such as "magnitude" and "hazard," into something tangible, so use simple language and check out their understanding.

Of course, your children's understanding will change and grow as they do; what you want to do is engage them and make preparedness the normal, natural response to possible disaster. This will give them the practical and psychological tools to survive an earthquake—and any number of other anxiety-provoking situations.

Learn to Manage Anxiety
Children and teens often need help recognizing that they feel anxious. Anxiety tends to announce itself through physical symptoms—often a stomach ache or headache—and critical thoughts such as "I'm weird" or "I'm going crazy." It's important to help your child become aware of these signs and to identify anxious feelings when they arise.

Do not fear that talking about anxiety will make your child more anxious. By explaining that we all experience anxiety you'll reduce any sense of isolation and shame.

Reassurance is key. Take children's fears and concerns seriously rather than dismissing them with a cheery "Don't worry! Relax!" By listening and showing empathy you can help your child open up and accept some guidance, and—this is especially important for teenagers—provide an opportunity to think out loud. Teach children and teens specific skills to help with anxiety, and remind them (and yourself) that anxiety isn't necessarily a bad thing—anxiety helps us prepare for danger.

> **Calm breathing and bubble blowing.** When you feel anxious, your breathing may change. Without being aware of it, you may take short, quick, shallow breaths or you may even hyperventilate. This can make the feeling of anxiety worse. Calm breathing is one technique you can use to deal with anxiety. It can be done with children of all ages and in a variety of stressful situations. Essentially, you become aware of your breathing, and then slow it down until you have regained a sense of control. Remind children they can use this technique when they are afraid or anxious, even if you are not there to help them. Practise calm breathing with your children using the following instructions:

1. Take a deep, slow breath in through your nose.

2. Breathe in deeply for four seconds.

3. Hold your breath for one or two seconds.

4. Breathe out slowly through your mouth.

5. Wait a few seconds before taking another breath.

6. Repeat for at least five breaths and for as many as ten breaths.

Bubble blowing can be helpful when teaching younger children how to do calm breathing. Using a homemade or commercial soap solution and a bubble wand (available at any toy store), have your child practise blowing bubbles. The slow exhaling required for making bubbles— especially when blowing a large bubble—is the same as for calm breathing. Make sure your child waits a second or two before blowing each bubble, and inhales slowly through the nose. Afterwards, practise this style of breathing without the bubble wand so that the child understands the bubbles aren't necessary for calm breathing.

> **Balloon belly breathing.** Children and adults can also benefit from the balloon belly breathing technique. Practise with your children using the following instructions:

1. Pretend that your belly is a balloon and you are blowing it up.

2. Breathe in deeply and fill (inflate) your balloon belly.

3. Slowly breathe out and empty (deflate) your balloon belly.

4. Try to keep your upper body (shoulders and chest) relaxed and still so that only your belly moves.

As with all emergency preparedness skills, building muscle memory is important. In order for you and your children to use breathing techniques effectively in an emergency situation, you should practise at least twice a day initially, doing ten calm breaths in a row. Practise when you are relaxed and not feeling anxious. Once you and your children are comfortable with these techniques, you can use them in any situations that cause anxiety.

EARTHQUAKE LEGENDS
FROM AROUND THE WORLD

Different cultures have explained earthquakes in different ways.

INDIA: The Earth is held up by four elephants that stand on the back of a turtle. The turtle is balanced on top of a cobra. When any of these animals move, the Earth trembles and shakes.

MEXICO: El Diablo, the devil, makes giant rips in the Earth from the inside. He and his devilish friends use the cracks when they want to come and stir up trouble on Earth.

SIBERIA: The Earth rests on a sled driven by a god named Tuli. The dogs who pull the sled have fleas. When they stop to scratch, the Earth shakes.

JAPAN: A great catfish, or *namazu*, lies curled up under the sea, with the islands of Japan resting on his back. A demigod, or *daimyojin*, holds a heavy stone over his head to keep *namazu* from moving. Once in a while, though, the *daimyojin* is distracted, the *namazu* moves, and the Earth trembles.

WEST AFRICA: The Earth is a flat disk, held up on one side by an enormous mountain and on the other by a giant. The giant's wife holds up the sky. The Earth trembles when he stops to hug her.

SCANDINAVIA: As punishment for murdering his brother, the god Loki is tied to a rock in an underground cave. Above his face is a serpent dripping poison, which Loki's sister catches in a bowl. From time to time, she has to go away to empty the bowl and the poison falls on Loki's face. He twists and wiggles to avoid it, and the ground shakes up above him.

NEW ZEALAND: Mother Earth has a child within her womb, the young god Ru. When he stretches and kicks as babies do, he causes earthquakes.

EAST AFRICA: A giant fish carries a stone on his back. A cow stands on the stone, balancing the Earth on one of her horns. From time to time, her neck begins to ache, and she tosses the globe from one horn to the other.

three

WEEK 1: GETTING STARTED
BEFORE AN EARTHQUAKE STRIKES

IN WEEK 1 of the readiness program you'll focus on two main tasks: developing an emergency communication plan and starting your home emergency kit. To develop your plan, you'll need to set aside twenty to sixty minutes, depending on the number of people in your household. To start your kit, you'll need more time, but much of the preparation can be done in combination with other regular shopping and household chores. Also, it is likely that you already have many of the items needed on hand and can simply add them to your kit.

Overview of Week 1 Steps

· Develop an emergency communication plan.

· Fill in a contact card for each member of your household.

· Start your home emergency kit, beginning with the essentials: water and food.

Keep yourself on track as you prepare during week 1 by using the checklist on page 125.

Emergency Communication Plan

Ask any disaster relief expert about the most important thing you can do to prepare for an earthquake and they'll tell you: Develop a plan. Along with gathering supplies, planning how you will respond when an earthquake hits is essential. A plan will help you perform better under stress, and build the real confidence—the resilience—you'll needed during a crisis.

Questions to Guide Planning

The goal of the emergency communication plan is to make sure all household members know what they should do to stay in touch.

Below is a list of questions that will take you through the points you want to cover in your plan. The questions are designed to allow you and those planning with you to think about likely emergency scenarios. Each household member should think through what might need to be done when disaster strikes. Children and teens in particular will benefit from being given the time to think out loud until the information makes sense to them. Try just to listen as they work things out. You can offer any necessary suggestions and corrections after giving children this chance to think and express their thoughts.

One way to begin the planning meeting (especially with children) is to say, "This week we are going to make a plan together so that if an earthquake happens we will know what to do and how to get in touch with family and friends. I'm going to ask some questions and we'll take turns answering them."

As you plan, you can make notes in whatever way suits you (on paper or an electronic device) and then summarize your decisions using the Emergency Communication Plan form on pages 126–127.

> **If an earthquake happens and we are not all together in the same place, how will we get in touch with each other?** You will need to establish your *non-local emergency contacts*. After an earthquake the local phones may go down or will likely be overloaded (as has happened in many emergency situations including recent ones in New Zealand and Japan) but it may be possible to make long-distance calls. It may not be possible to talk on cell phones because of tower damage or system overload, but it may be possible to send text messages.

Your non-local emergency contacts will usually be relatives or friends who live outside the affected area—and ideally outside of your own city or region—who can be contacted by all family members if it becomes impossible to reach home or reunion sites. Everyone should know to text, call, or email the same person. Have a backup person as well. For example, "First we'll call Uncle Carl. If he's not home we'll contact Aunt Joyce."

> **Where will we meet after an earthquake?** You will need to establish your *reunion sites*. You may or may not be with your family when an earthquake strikes, and there's a good chance that all members of your household will not be at home. Where will you meet and how will you find each other? Talk about possible locations and come up with two or three sites in your neighbourhood where you could meet after an earthquake. You should have a primary site and a couple of secondary sites as backup in case the primary site is not accessible. Consider meeting at a local school, park, church, or community centre. Household members who leave home should write a note telling others where they have gone. Pick a place to leave this note, either near the front door or in an obvious location outside.

> **How will we remember this information and keep in contact?** You will need to fill out a *contact card* (page 128) for each person in your household. Adults can keep their contact cards in a wallet and in digital form in their electronic devices. School-aged children can tape their contact cards inside a binder or notebook or put them in a lunch box, book bag, or wallet. You can have as many copies of each contact card as you want—the important thing is to have the information accessible in an emergency.

> **What will we do if we are away from home—at school or at work?** You will need to discuss all the possible arrangements that might be required depending on where everyone is. This is a good opportunity to hear from children about any emergency plans discussed at school. All schools have emergency plans, and most schools on the west coast of North America have earthquake plans. If you find your child has no idea about a school emergency plan, this is a cue to talk with a teacher or principal.

Let children know that the most important thing is to find a safe place. Help them remember where these places are at school. Remind them to follow the directions from their teacher or principal and to stay calm.

> **What else do we need to talk about?** You will need to make other plans based on where you live and what the members of your household do. You might live in an urban or a rural area, in a condo or a house. Household members might be very young or very old or have physical or mental disabilities. You might have a dog or a cat. Later chapters will cover safety considerations for those with special needs (Chapter 5) and for pets (Chapter 6).

> **When should we revisit our plan?** You will need to set a date to look at your plan again as your household circumstances change over time.

Tips for Children

Make sure you include children of all ages in planning. Ask them to contribute their ideas and give them opportunities to be resourceful. Asking teenagers and older children to take notes at your planning meeting is a good way to give them a role and involve them.

Prepare for Communication Challenges

Be prepared to have communication networks fail in the immediate aftermath of an earthquake. Cell phones, cordless and regular phones connected to land lines, computers, and the many hand-held devices we've come to depend upon may not work, and you may be without a communication device for days and possibly longer. Keep your cell or smart phone with you just in case you are able to call or send a text message after an earthquake, but know that even if you do send a tweet or a text, you may need to wait for days before emergency personnel arrive. Also keep in mind that powering your computer or recharging the batteries for any electronic device may present challenges.

> **Create a printed copy of your entire phone list.** I know from recent power outage experiences that you cannot get the phone numbers of friends and family from your cordless phone memory without electricity. Even if you have many contact numbers in your cell phone, it would be good to reserve your phone's battery for an emergency.

> **Put ICE (In Case of Emergency) in front of the name of your emergency contact person in your cell phone.** This will make it easier for you to find the number, and if you lose your phone or are injured, this will allow someone else to reach your emergency contact person.

> **Prepare children for overloaded communication networks.** Reassure children and teens that it may take some time to

get through on any phone after an earthquake. Tell them to keep trying.

> **Send a text message rather than making a voice call.** In major emergencies, such as 9/11 and the Japanese 2011 quake, the phone networks were overwhelmed as everyone tried to reach their loved ones at the same moment. A text message uses far less bandwidth than a voice call, which means you will have a greater likelihood of getting through with a text, and you will be freeing voice lines for emergency service use.

> **Adjust your expectations of social media.** The use of social media such as Facebook and Twitter during recent disasters in Haiti, New Zealand, and Japan marks a major shift in disaster response. Immediately following the quake in Haiti, Facebook received over fifteen hundred status updates per minute and the earthquake became the top topic on Twitter.

The disaster response community, however, was unprepared for this onslaught of information and since then has been strategizing about how they can keep up with the overwhelming mass of information streaming online during a disaster.

To find out about social media use and expectations, the American Red Cross conducted an online survey in the summer of 2010, asking adults how they would try to contact emergency services if they needed help and couldn't access 9-1-1. One in five respondents said they would turn to digital means such as email or Twitter for help. But what was most revealing was the unrealistic expectations of these survey-takers.

More than fifty percent believed (wrongly) that an agency of some kind monitors and responds to urgent requests on Twitter and Facebook. Seventy-four percent expected help to arrive within an hour after a tweet or Facebook post, while twenty-eight percent expected help to arrive within fifteen minutes. Although social media will continue to play a role in emergencies, you would be wise not to expect these impossibly speedy responses.

> **Consider some low-tech communication alternatives.** Japan is perhaps the most technologically advanced country in the world. For many, the loss of instant connection following the 2011 earthquake was almost as terrifying as the quake itself. "When cell phones went down, there was paralysis and panic," said Shoji Ogasawara, the head of emergency communications at Miyako's city hall. "Everyone was running around asking, 'What happened to the nuclear plant? What happened to our town?'"

While many found their inability to send texts or check online messages an eerily lonely experience—"I felt so isolated," lamented one seventeen-year-old, "You don't realize how much you rely on something until you lose it"—others turned to old-school, low-tech communication methods to find news of loved ones. People relied on newspapers, radio, and even lists of names on paper notices. One shop near the Fukushima nuclear plant had hundreds of people descending on it daily, looking for newspapers with lists of names of local people who had been found or rescued. Areas waiting for cell phone service to be restored relied on a makeshift emergency radio station, newsletters put out by a local refugee centre, and even a network of outdoor loudspeakers dating back to World War II.

Practise Your Plan
After you have summarized your plan in written form and filled out your contact cards, take the next step and

practise some aspects of your plan. For instance, you might visit your reunion sites with family members by walking to each location from home. You might then try taking different routes to your reunion sites from various key locations in your neighbourhood.

When I was a kid, I knew my way around a large portion of the city I lived in because we walked everywhere. Today this isn't necessarily the case—we tend to drive our kids almost everywhere. This puts them at a disadvantage should an earthquake occur when we aren't with them. Do what you can to overcome this. For instance, when you are shopping or at a soccer game with your children, practise getting to your reunion site from the store or sports field.

Start Your Home Emergency Kit

The mantra in the Earthquake preparedness field is "Be ready for seventy-two hours." This means that we need to prepare ourselves to make it through the first three days—seventy-two hours—after a disaster without any outside help. Of course, this is the minimum amount of time; some experts believe it is more realistic to aim for seven days of self-sufficiency.

After an earthquake, rescue professionals will be busy trying to save lives and move emergency equipment, medicine, and supplies to the hardest-hit areas. Because you may not see any first-responders for several days, you will need to have water and a container with food and various supplies.

What kind of container is best for a home emergency kit? This is simple: whatever will hold the food and supplies your household needs. My family uses a large plastic container we found at the local hardware store. A brand new metal or plastic garbage can with a tight-fitting lid works well if you have space in a garage or shed. A waterproof container is a good idea.

Where to Store Your Kit
When picking a storage location for your kit, consider finding somewhere cool, dry, and protected from direct sunlight and freezing temperatures. Ideally, you want an easily accessed location close to a main exit. If you live in an apartment you might want to put the kit on bricks and a board in the back of a closet. Wherever you store your kit, be sure to do the following:

- Label the kit with the date packed and the last date reviewed.

- Keep the kit off the floor where it can be safe from flooding and protected from insects and other critters.

- Keep the kit away from walls, especially concrete ones, to prevent heat and condensation from affecting the contents.

What to Include
At the end of the four-week readiness program, your emergency kit will contain what you need to manage on your own for at least seventy-two hours, including:

- Water

- Food

- Essential medications and personal toiletries

- First aid kit

- Flashlight and radio with extra batteries

- Tent or tarp

- Small stove and fuel

- Sleeping bags

- Cooking and eating utensils

- Tools, including a wrench for turning off gas and water

- Supplies such as toilet paper, garbage bags, duct tape, and bleach

You do not have to assemble the kit contents all at once. You can add to your equipment and supplies over time. Once your kit is assembled you can relax and ignore it, with one exception: you'll need to rotate your water supply and food every six months. This may sound like a lot of work, but it's not. Make a note in your calendar when you need to change. Many people use the change from standard time to daylight savings time and back again. When the day selected arrives, water containers can be refreshed and cans of food can be used or donated to the local food bank. If you have teenagers, this is a great job for them (of course, you will want to give them a reminder and you may need to provide some help).

Store Water
Next to air, water is the most necessary substance for human survival. You can survive for weeks without food, but can only go without water for a few days. After an earthquake, access to water—whether you rely on a public system or a private well—may be severely limited or completely cut off.

You will need to keep a three-day supply of water on hand for each member of your household. This will be used for drinking, cooking, and personal hygiene. Don't forget to include water for your pets and extra water for any household member with special needs (an elderly person, a nursing mother, or someone who is ill).

Start with 4 litres (1 gallon) per person per day. This means each person will need at least 12 litres (3 gallons) for the seventy-two hours. To get a picture of this, think of the commercial containers of water you have seen used in an office or home water cooler. The most common size is just under 20 litres (roughly 5 gallons). For a family of three, you could pick up two of these containers and you'd be covered for the seventy-two hours. You could also store eighteen 2-litre (0.5-gallon) soft drink bottles and you would have enough water for three days. Whatever quantity of water you store, keep it in a cool, dark place.

Containers
The top-of-the-line containers are stainless steel. The main advantage is that you can store a large amount of water for a long time and it will taste better than water stored in plastic. The drawback is that stainless containers can be expensive. You can also use water barrels with an attached pump. I often think I'd like to get one of those; perhaps someday if I count my pennies.

Plastic containers are usually cheap, light, and recyclable, and you can buy stackable kinds. However, there are health concerns with certain grades of plastic. Avoid containers marked with the number 3 recycling symbol. Be sure to use food-grade plastic storage containers. Note that reusing plastic milk jugs is not recommended because milk protein is hard to remove and can cause bacterial growth in stored water.

As mentioned above, you can reuse 2-litre soft drink bottles. Although the plastic in these can outgas, which means break down and leach as vapour into the water, this can be avoided by storing the bottles in a cool, dark place. Putting the bottles in a black plastic garbage bag is one easy way to keep out the light.

Many disaster preparation guides do not recommended glass bottles for the obvious reason that they can break. Despite this danger, and even with the added disadvantage of glass being heavier than plastic, this is what we use at our house. Why? Because we had large apple cider bottles on hand, and because I trust that glass won't break down and poison the water. This works for us because we have the space to store big glass bottles, but if they break I'm sure I'll wish I'd used other containers.

In any case, start with the container choice that means you will get the job done. You can always reassess and make changes at one of your regular six-month rotation dates.

How to Clean and Fill Your Containers
Thoroughly clean the containers with dishwashing soap and water, and rinse completely so there is no residual soap. Sanitize each container with a solution of unscented liquid household chlorine bleach (5 millilitres bleach to 1 litre water or 1 teaspoon bleach to 1 quart water). Swish the sanitizing solution in the container so that it touches all surfaces. After sanitizing, thoroughly rinse out the bleach solution with clean water.

Keep it simple: tap water is the easiest and best to use. Most municipal water has been treated for bacteria already. If you use well water like I do, remember that it hasn't been treated with chlorine so you'll need to add one drop of unscented bleach to each litre or quart of water. Close the container tightly, being careful not to contaminate the cap by touching the inside with your finger. Be sure to label the containers with the date they were filled.

Some people store their water in a cool, dark corner of the garage or basement. Under a sink works well too—just be sure not to store plastic next to toxic substances such as paint thinner, gas, or cleaning supplies. The fumes can leach into plastic and contaminate the water.

If you are using plastic, put some bottles in your freezer. A full freezer runs more efficiently and it's another source of water in an emergency. Make sure you leave some room for the water to expand as it freezes. Make six-month notes in your calendar to replace the water. You can also just keep rotating through your bottles by using them to water your plants.

Other Sources of Emergency Water

If for some reason you can't get to your emergency water supply, or if it runs out (or if your glass bottles break), there are other sources of water to be found in your home. A hot water tank can supply 30 to 60 litres (6 to 12 gallons) in an emergency. You can also use melted ice cubes and the liquid from canned fruit and vegetables. Another water source is your toilet tank. This one I admit makes me a bit squeamish, but if I was out of water, I'm sure I'd soon get over it. You need to purify this water first by adding unscented bleach.

Store Food

There is a wealth of information available about which foods last and which keep their nutritional value the longest. Just remember—it's better to have some food put away then to spend your valuable time researching which packaged survival foods are best. Buy and assemble the things you and your family members will be happy to eat—probably the same things that you pick up on a regular grocery shopping trip.

Containers

Use food-grade containers for storing anything you intend to eat. A food-grade container is one that contains no chemicals that are hazardous to human health and will not transfer undesirable tastes and odours into the food.

Avoid canned food and drink containers with pop-top lids. These lids can leak or allow the container to explode.

Keep dry foods in airtight, moisture-proof containers away from direct light and heat. Store packaged food (crackers, cereal, etc.) in resealable plastic bags, airtight plastic food storage containers, or glass jars with screw-top lids. These bags and containers can then be used for storing the opened packages and keeping the food fresh as you use it.

Type of Food

Canned and dried foods are the staples in any home emergency kit. Again, you will want enough food for three days for each member of your household. Assume you will need the equivalent of half a 398-millilitre (14-ounce) can per person for each meal. A family of three will need four and a half cans per day or thirteen and a half cans for seventy-two hours.

While you can invest in specially prepared survival foods, you can also just use what you eat on a regular basis. The simplest choice for your kit is commercially canned food.

> **Dried foods.** As any hiker knows, dried or dehydrated foods hold their nutrition, last a long time, take up little space, are light to carry, and are easy to prepare. And also as any hiker knows, you need to buy them at an outdoor equipment store and add spices to make them more palatable.

> MRES. Short for *meals, ready-to-eat,* these are prepared meals in lightweight ration packages used by the military.

They come with utensils and can be heated by placing the whole package in hot water. These are among the easiest of foods, but MRES are expensive (usually $8 to $10 a meal). You can buy these at an army surplus store and online.

> **Commercially canned foods.** The food is already cooked and can be eaten right out of the can. How long will canned food last? In general, home-canned foods should be eaten within a year. Commercially canned low-acid foods last the longest (I read an astonishing story about a can of meat opened after 118 years that was found to have retained most of its nutrients). However, the usual recommendation is to eat the food in two to five years. Canned fruit, tomatoes, and anything with a lot of vinegar is best used within a year. These foods may last longer than a year but their taste and nutritional value will decline.

The bottom line? Think about what you and your family like to eat and take the shopping list provided on page 129 with you the next time you go to the supermarket. Once you buy and store your emergency food in a cool, dry place along with your water, you'll be set.

Week 1 Summary

Complete your preparations with the help of these checklists and forms found at the end of this book:

· Week 1 Checklist

· Emergency Communication Plan

· Contact Card

· Shopping List for Home Emergency Kit

FIVE REASONS TO PREPARE
FOR AN EARTHQUAKE

1. You want to keep your family safe. Preparing will reduce
   the risk of injury in the event of an earthquake.

2. You want to set a good example for your children. Incorporating
   preparedness into the culture of your family will teach your
   children about dealing with practical and psychological
   challenges. What a great legacy!

3. You want to be able to help others. Being prepared will put you in
   a good position to support others in your neighbourhood and local
   community.

4. You want to cover your financial bases. Having a plan in place
   will ensure the least amount of damage to your home and
   property.

5. You want to feel less anxious. Knowing that you have made plans
   and are ready to act will lower your anxiety level about earthquakes and other emergencies.

four

WEEK 2: PREPARING YOURSELF AND YOUR HOME

IN WEEK 2 of the readiness program you'll make some simple changes to your home that will prevent the most common cause of injury in an earthquake: falling household objects. You'll also add to the home emergency kit that you started in week 1.

Overview of Week 2 Steps
· Identify hazards in your home.

· Eliminate hazards.

· Complete your home emergency kit.

Keep yourself on track as you prepare during week 2 by using the checklist on page 130.

Identify Earthquake Hazards
We know from past experience that it is the contents of our homes—our furniture, appliances, dishes, ornaments, and other items—that are most often damaged and cause the

most preventable harm in an earthquake. When our homes shake, bookcases topple and cupboard doors fly open, releasing all kinds of objects and sending them through the air. The good news is that we can reduce the risk of being struck by falling objects and prevent damage to our homes and their contents with some simple preparation.

Begin by gathering the supplies you will need to assess your home for hazards:

- A piece of plain paper or graph paper for drawing a floor plan

- A pencil or coloured pencils

- The Earthquake Hazard Hunt form (pages 131–133)

Prepare a rough drawing of your home's floor plan or ask a member of your household to do this. Next, walk through your home with household members and look for furniture and other objects at risk of falling or breaking in an earthquake.

If you live in an apartment building or condo, your hazard hunt might involve touring some of the shared spaces, such as the lobby or laundry room, with fellow tenants or neighbours. Whether you live in an apartment or a single-family dwelling, participating in this kind of an assessment will give you an opportunity to connect with and discuss preparation with those most likely to be with you when an earthquake strikes—your family members, roommates, and neighbours. It's also a wonderful opportunity to talk with children, to find out what they already know or what they've picked up from school or online, and to help reduce everyone's anxiety by making immediate changes that will most definitely reduce your risk of injury.

Potential Perils

As you walk through each room in your home, see if there are any of the following objects or potentially dangerous situations and make notes about them on your floor plan and form:

- Heavy or fragile objects on high shelves

- Wall-mounted pictures, TV sets, mirrors, or clocks

- Hanging lights, plants, or other heavy objects

- Rolling carts holding a TV or other heavy object

- Beds placed under or beside a large window

- Electronic equipment or small appliances on high open shelves, desktops, or countertops

- Bookshelves and other open shelf units

- Cabinets and cupboards with doors that might fly open

- Unsecured tall appliances and heavy furniture

- Gas stove with an inflexible feed line

- Unsecured hot water tank

Tips for Children

The hazard hunt can be an especially good way to involve children in preparedness tasks. Sketching—and colouring—the floor plan you will use can be a good job for some children, and even young children can take part in a hazard hunt using a list of potential perils with pictures added. As the child finds each item, you can explain the danger presented by the object or situation and how you will handle this. You might award points for each item a child finds, and give a prize or plan a special outing for the winner.

Secure Your Belongings

Once you have identified the hazards in your home, immediately eliminate those that you can:

> **Heavy or fragile objects.** Move any objects that could
> become dangerous projectiles, including plants in break-
> able pots and metal or glass items, from high to lower
> shelves or to the inside of latched cabinets.

> **Electronic equipment and small appliances.** Move computer
> monitors, printers, TVs, microwaves, and toasters from
> high to lower surfaces.

> **Wall-mounted and hanging objects, especially when above
> a bed or couch.** Move any objects that cannot be securely
> attached to a wall, ceiling, or a shelf. If you want to leave
> pictures in place, pinch the backs of standard picture-
> hanging hooks so that they close over the picture wire and
> ensure the pictures won't "jump" off the wall when the
> shaking starts, and be sure to install picture hooks directly
> into the wall studs.

> **Rolling carts holding heavy objects.** Lock cart wheels.

> **Beds placed under or beside a large window.** Move any beds
> away from windows or cover windows with heavy blinds or
> curtains.

To eliminate some hazards, you will need more time as well
as some tools and materials. Make a plan to tackle these,
perhaps on a room-by-room basis:

> **Objects you do not want to move or cannot move.** Use
> products available at office supply and hardware stores to
> attach items securely to shelves, counters, and walls. Strips

of Velcro with adhesive on the back can be cut into squares to hold larger items in place. A reusable adhesive product can also be used to secure items. This product comes in putty or gel form and is sold under various names, including museum wax and earthquake wax. You just mash it with your fingers and stick it between the item and the surface. This works on the underside of pottery or dishes, and doesn't remove the paint or finish the way Velcro strips can. Another option is double-sided transparent or foam tape, which can be purchased in rolls and individual pieces. Both sides are sticky, and although the adhesive can smudge the surface and object you are securing, an oil-based furniture polish will usually remove the residue.

> **Electronic equipment and small appliances at risk of falling**. Secure these items with slip-proof mats, rug pads (the kind you use under throw rugs to keep them in place), or rubberized drawer liners.

> **Open shelf units**. Use straps or guardrails to prevent objects—particularly glass objects—from sliding off.

> **Bookshelves, tall appliances, and heavy furniture**. Secure loaded bookshelves, tall appliances such as refrigerators and stacked washer-dryer units, and free-standing furniture using flexible-mount fasteners with nylon straps. These allow the appliance or furniture to move independently from the wall. Note that in the past many people (including me) secured their furniture and appliances with metal L-brackets. Even though these are no longer considered the best way to secure tall and heavy items, they do work and I will probably not change mine. Whatever method you use, secure the top right and left corners and make sure you are screwing into the wall studs not just into the drywall.

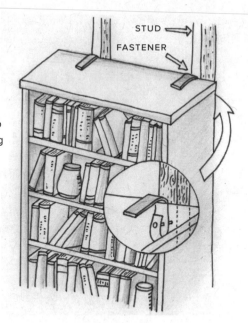

STUD

FASTENER

Flexible fasteners allow tall objects to sway without falling over, reducing the strain on the studs.

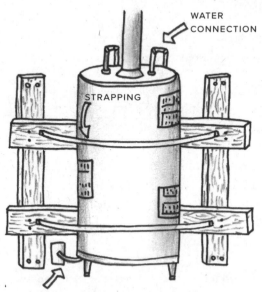

WATER CONNECTION

STRAPPING

Bracing a hot water tank prevents it from falling over and rupturing the attached water and gas or electricity lines.

GAS OR ELECTRICITY CONNECTION

> **Cabinets and cupboards.** Look at all the doors in the kitchen, bathrooms, and bedrooms to ensure the latches will hold. If you don't think they will hold under the stress of an earthquake, replace them or add additional fasteners designed for this purpose.

> **Gas stove.** If your gas stove has a rigid rather than a flexible gas line, arrange to have the line upgraded.

> **Hot water tank.** Use sheet-metal strapping to secure your tank to the wall. This is worth paying a tradesperson to do if you don't feel up to the task.

Complete Your Home Emergency Kit

In week 1 you started assembling your home emergency kit by storing some water and food; now it's time to add the other essential supplies that will help you survive the first seventy-two hours after an earthquake or any other disaster.

Review the Home Emergency Kit Supplies list on pages 134–135 to determine what items you already have on hand (cooking and eating utensils, aluminum foil) and what you might need to buy (up-to-date first aid book, windup radio). Heavy-duty garbage bags and duct tape are both essential supplies that have a number of uses. For instance, garbage bags can be used to make a rain poncho or shelter, while duct tape can be used to repair shoes and gear, temporarily waterproof items, and add a reflective coating to an emergency signaling device. A pair of work gloves is another good item for your home emergency kit (and your car emergency kit), since you will very likely find yourself needing to move debris and clean up broken glass. A whistle, too, is good to include so that you can signal for help.

In addition to the essential supplies listed, you might consider adding the following to your kit:

- Water purification tablets
- Basic tool kit—hammer, pliers, multipurpose screwdrivers, etc.
- Needle and thread
- Plastic bucket with lid (can be lined with a garbage bag and used in lieu of a loo)
- Signal flare
- "Help" sign
- Protective masks and goggles
- Two-storey emergency escape ladder (This relatively inexpensive item can be stored compactly under a bed on an upper floor.)

Week 2 Summary
Complete your preparations with the help of these check-lists and forms found at the end of the book:

- Week 2 Checklist
- Earthquake Hazard Hunt
- Home Emergency Kit Supplies

THE OMINOUS ROLL OF THE EARTHQUAKE

In Sara Dean's early-twentieth-century novel of crime and redemption, *Travers: A Story of the San Francisco Earthquake,* a woman confronts an intruder in her home just as the 1906 quake strikes. It is not known whether Dean experienced the earthquake herself or merely fashioned her story out of contemporary accounts. Either way, her detailed and frightening description shows why you want to secure the objects in your home.

But Nature now took her hand in this strange interview. Two sharp detonations sounded like the booming of artillery. A second later and the whole room vibrated, suddenly, with a sort of sullen determination. The chandelier swung violently, scattering the globes afar. Gwen's dressing table tottered, danced forward, bowed and fell, hurling its burden of silver and glass in all directions. The bookcase advanced a few feet into the room, then capsized, scattering a rain of volumes. The clock and two tall vases on the mantelpiece began a strange jig-reeling, drawing nearer to one another, retreating, bowing and becking in Bacchanalian fashion. The windows rattled madly in their casings as if shaken by a frenzied hand, then sash by sash, the glass shivered.

Gwendolyn clung to her brass bedstead. It was moving from side to side with a violent motion that threatened to throw her out upon the floor. The burglar reeled and grasped the foot of the bed for support, took a step and lunged with a heavy roll against the wall nearby. At the same moment a picture above him fell with a heavy crash.

Around and about sounded the jarring rush of falling brick.

The shrill screams of the servants on the floor above reached Gwendolyn's ears; and then gradually the fact stole over her consciousness that beneath and pervading all the scattered many-voiced pandemonium of sounds was the long, hollow, subterranean rumble, constant, deepening, but never ceasing—the ominous roll of the Earthquake...

A beam crushed through the ceiling above her head—then another. The writhing, jarring earth seemed to renew its fury and take on an added determination to annihilate. A rain of bricks began to pour into the room upon the bed, upon Gwendolyn.

Without a word the burglar flung himself toward her, sheltering her with his broad shoulders, deflecting the flying missiles as best he could. The air was full of mortar. His hands closed over her mouth, to keep out the floating, smothering grey powder.

The earth twisted, writhed, jarred on like a creature in torture; then suddenly all was still.

five

WEEK 3:
FINDING SAFE PLACES

IN WEEK 3 of the readiness program you'll practise the single most important way to respond when an earthquake strikes—drop, cover, and hold on. You'll do this a number of times in a variety of settings so that you are not tempted to run when the ground shakes. You'll then look for safe places to shelter during an earthquake. You'll also assemble a personal grab-and-go bag that contains identification, clothing, and other essentials. If necessary, you'll consider the safety of any household members who have special needs because of age or disability.

Overview of Week 3 Steps

· Rehearse drop, cover, and hold on.

· Look for safe places in your home and away from home.

· Assemble a personal grab-and-go bag for each member of your household.

· Consider any special needs of household members.

Keep yourself on track as you prepare during week 3 by using the checklist on page 136.

Rehearse Drop, Cover, and Hold On

Emergency professionals continue to recommend that you drop, cover, and hold on in response to an earthquake for very good reasons. See discussion on the "Triangle of Life" theory on page 102.

> **Drop.** You should drop to the ground and curl up so that you present as little surface area as possible for falling and flying objects to strike. Staying upright and trying to run away from the shaking of an earthquake exposes you to all kinds of risk, from falling down stairs to being struck by an airborne lamp.

> **Cover.** Once you've got yourself low to the ground, you should cover up. Get under a table or a desk. If that's impossible, move away from mirrors, windows, doors, and tall furniture. Pick a spot on an inside wall where there

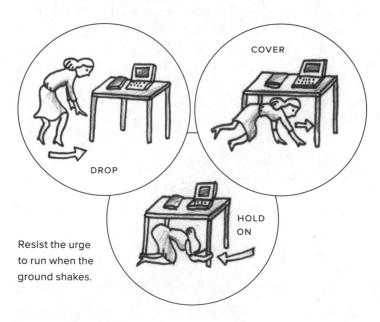

COVER

DROP

HOLD ON

Resist the urge to run when the ground shakes.

is nothing overhead. Crouch on the floor with your back to the wall. If possible, cover your head and neck with pillows, blankets, magazines, cushions off a chair or couch—anything you can reach that will protect you from flying shards of glass and other hazards.

> **Hold on.** While you are down and covered, you should old on to the biggest, most secure object you can find—the leg of a desk or table will do. Don't underestimate the power of an earthquake to fling you from one place to another.

Take a Safe-at-Home Tour

In the same way that you walked through your home looking for hazards, you now need to walk through looking for safe places to shelter. As you tour your home, pay attention to staircases, hallways, and all the other locations you might find yourself in when an earthquake strikes. You want to identify places where you might take shelter, as well as all the possible emergency exit and access points. Take the time to explore the options with household members. In each room and area, ask, "Where is the safest place to be if an earthquake happened right now?"

Remember that your first impulse will be to run outside. The fear will surge and your mind will scream "Go!" Remind everyone in your household why running outside is a bad idea:

· You will have only a few seconds to react and retreat to a safe place. Running outside will use up precious moments.

· You want to make yourself as small a target as possible for the objects that will fly through the air during an earthquake. Running will make you a large moving target.

- You are safest far away from the known dangers outside—falling power lines and building materials shaken from exteriors—masonry, window glass, bricks. Running will expose you to serious injury as objects rain down from above.

> **Should I stand in a doorway?** No. Experts used to think a doorway, protected by a door frame, was the safest place to be in an earthquake. This is no longer case. In fact, you're more likely to be hurt by a door slamming shut, by flying objects, or by other people hurrying to get out through the doorway.

> **What if I am in bed?** If you are in bed when a quake hits, the safest thing to do is to stay there, cover your head and neck with a pillow, and wait until the shaking has stopped. This can take from a few seconds to several minutes, and will seem like hours. It's a good idea to keep a pair of shoes under your bed so that you can safely move about after an earthquake. If you try to run barefoot from your bedroom, broken glass on the floor can cause serious injury. Once the shaking has stopped, take an extra few seconds and pull on your shoes.

> **What if my children are in another room?** Although you will naturally want to run to your children, wherever they are in your home, this is a flight response you should not give in to.

If you are in bed it is likely dark and the power may already be out. Even if it's light enough to see, if you get out of bed during a major earthquake you run the risk of being thrown to the ground or having a flying object injure you or knock you unconscious. This would make it difficult if not impossible to get to your children. Regardless of the circumstance, you and your children want to respond in

the same way—drop, cover, and hold on. Once the immediate threat of the earthquake has passed and you have
all survived the initial shake, you can go to your children,
review the situation, and start to think about what to
do next.

Extending the Tour

After you have toured your home and identified safe places,
continue looking for good spots to shelter when you are
away from home. When you go to the store or the park, and
when you're riding on public transit, get into the habit of
looking for safe places and exits.

Wherever you are when an earthquake happens—in
a school, an office building, or a parking lot—you should
drop, cover, and hold on. Remember that you should never
use elevators during or after an earthquake, and that
sprinkler systems and fire alarms are likely to be activated
by the shaking. Always avoid windows and other obvious
hazards, such as stacks of boxes in supermarkets or heavy
hanging signs.

If you are already outdoors, scan your surrounding for
potential hazards—power lines, trees, building facades—
and move to a clear area if you can safely do so. Otherwise
drop and cover your head and neck with your arms and
your jacket or whatever else you have on hand.

Tips for Children

Children will likely have many questions as you look
around your home and elsewhere for safe places to shelter
during an earthquake. Watch for subtle signs of anxiety,
especially a tendency to deny danger exists or persistent
requests to "get something to eat" or "watch a movie"—
anything other than prepare. Watch as well for more overt
expressions of fear and find ways to reassure children that

preparing for an emergency is the best way to relieve feelings of anxiety.

You might want to make a game of identifying safe places ("Am I in a safe place standing in this doorway?") or hold an actual earthquake drill. Yell "Earthquake!" and make sure everyone drops to the ground, crawls under a table or desk, and holds on tight. If there are pillows or other good shielding items within reach, encourage everyone to grab something and use it for head and neck protection.

You might also want to remind children what to do if they are in bed when an earthquake strikes. Have them practise covering their heads with pillows and ask them to repeat to you what they should do: "Stay in bed, pillow on head. Mom and Dad will come."

Assemble a Personal Grab-and-Go Bag

When disaster strikes, you will have very little time to act. In the event of fire, you will have about two minutes, and in the case of an earthquake, you will have seconds. What do you need? "Gathering" is one of those irrational behaviours that humans engage in during emergencies. Rather than heading for safety immediately, many people automatically start looking for objects to take with them. This can be the result of a "normalcy bias"—we stick to our routines, intent on finishing the email we're writing or the dishes we're washing, and assume we have the time to pack for leaving home in the same way we always do. This behaviour can also be the result of our inability to focus or think clearly as our bodies are flooded with adrenaline.

It's vital to remember that a few minutes of looking around and gathering random objects could cost you your life. Instead, you need to have something ready to walk out with at a moment's notice: a grab-and-go bag. Every household member should have a portable collection of important personal items, including identification, cash, and prescription medication.

Although you can buy prepackaged evacuation kits online or from stores, it's cheaper and better to assemble your own. A backpack is the most efficient kind of bag to use since it is easy to carry and the good ones are strong and roomy enough to hold what you need. Use whatever bag you have at home—an old backpack, a small duffle bag, a cast-off book bag. You can go to a store at a later date and buy a light, waterproof, durable bag if you want to, but remember the point is to get ready now. You can always upgrade your bag later.

After you have found or bought a bag for each member of your household, use the Personal Grab-and-Go Bag Supplies list on pages 137–139 to assemble what you will need:

· Identification

· Cash (bank machines are likely to be down after an earthquake and it may not be possible to use credit cards everywhere)

· Clothing

· Snacks and water

· Toiletries and medication

· Emergency blanket (available from stores that carry camping supplies)

· Family and pet photos

Keep children and teens involved in the preparedness process by having them assemble their own bags. With your guidance and the supplies list, they can gather many of the items needed.

Consider Safety for Infants

If you have an infant, you will want to practise dropping, covering, and holding on with the baby in your arms. You will also need to include additional supplies in both your home emergency kit and your baby's grab-and-go bag. If your baby is bottle fed or is just being introduced to solid food, you will want to make sure that your kit includes some formula and canned or jarred baby food. You will also want to include bedding, bottles, and disposable diapers. If your baby is breastfed, it is a good idea to include extra fluids for yourself and some emergency formula in case you have trouble with your milk supply—sometimes stressful situations and limited food and water intake can reduce the amount of milk you produce.

Your baby's personal grab-and-go bag will not need most of the items included in an adult or child's bag. Instead, your baby's bag should contain formula, food, diapers, clothes (more than you would pack for an adult or child), and baby wipes. You might also include the following items:

- Baby shampoo, powder, and lotion

- Vitamins

- Medicine dropper

- Nasal aspirator

- Sunscreen

- Toys

Consider Safety for Seniors and People with Disabilities

If you are a senior or have a disability (or help care for someone who does), you may wish to make some additional plans for an emergency. ·

If you are not able to use stairs or have other mobility problems, be prepared to stay in a safe place until help comes. Think about installing plug-in security lights. These will stay lit for several hours after a power outage and can provide the illumination needed during what may be a slower or more difficult evacuation process. If you use life-support equipment that requires electricity, think about getting a small generator as a backup power source. Also consider arranging for a buddy—a neighbour or nearby friend or relative—to provide additional support during an emergency. Share with your buddy whatever he or she needs to know about your physical limitations or disability. Include your buddy's name, phone number, and address in your emergency communication plan. Give your buddy a copy of your home's floor plan with notes about obstacles, exits, and alternate escape routes.

If you use a walker or cane, consider having a backup walker or cane in another part of your home. If you use a wheelchair and are in the chair when an earthquake strikes, stay in the chair, set the brake, and cover your head with one arm while holding the chair with the other.

In addition to the standard supplies included in a personal grab-and-go bag, make sure your bag contains:

- A description of your medical condition, allergies, and any special dietary requirements

- A list of all the medications you take

- Your doctor's name and phone number

Week 3 Summary

Complete your preparations with the help of these check-lists found at the end of the book:

- Week 3 Checklist
- Personal Grab-and-Go Bag Supplies

EARTHQUAKES IN MUSIC AND ART

All kinds of artists, inspired by the power and mystery of earthquakes, have been moved to create concertos, paintings, installations, and interpretive dance pieces.

In 1855, after a major earthquake damaged Edo, Japan (present-day Tokyo), artists produced woodblock prints depicting both the destruction and the "cause"—a mythical giant catfish (*namazu*) thrashing about in their underground lairs. Many buyers believed the prints offered protection against future earthquakes.

More recently, U.S. Geological Survey seismologist and trombone player Andrew Michael turned earthquake waves into music. Michael's quartet for trombone, cello, voice, and seismogram is a thunderous, jazzy piece based on speeded-up audio recordings of a quake. Michael chose instruments he felt could suggest the quality of seismic waves and relied especially on the cello, he says, because "the way a cello bow sticks and slips against the strings is similar to some of the ideas we have about how faults stick and slip."

---

six

WEEK 4: STAYING SAFE IN THE CAR AND AT WORK

IN WEEK 4 of the readiness program you'll prepare to stay safe when you are away from home, either travelling in your car or spending time at your workplace. You'll also consider making a plan for your pets and will review what you've done so far and might still need to do to get ready for an earthquake.

Overview of Week 4 Steps

· Assemble a car emergency kit.

· Assemble a work emergency kit.

· Assemble a pet emergency kit.

· Review preparations made so far.

Keep yourself on track as you prepare during week 4 by using the checklist on page 140.

Stay Safe in the Car

An earthquake could happen while you are returning from work or when you're on your way to the grocery store. You could be on a bridge, a busy highway, or a quiet rural road. Wherever you drive, you need to prepare for this possibility in two ways:

1. Make sure you have emergency supplies in your car.

2. Know how to control your car when the ground shakes.

Keeping Your Car Ready

First of all, it's a good idea to keep your gas tank as full as possible at all times. Not only is this the most efficient way to run your car, it will ensure you have fuel after an emergency occurs. Remember that gas stations may not be able to operate for some time after a major earthquake. Next, you need to assemble a car emergency kit—this will be a great resource during any kind of emergency, including a side-of-the-highway breakdown. Chances are, you already have many of the items in your car (booster cables, first aid, kit) and will only need to add some food and water to be ready. See the Car Emergency Kit Supplies list on pages 141–142.

Driving in an Earthquake

Driving during a major quake is extremely difficult and dangerous. You may feel as though your car is a boat at sea being pushed from underneath by strong waves, and at the same time as though you have one or several flat tires—your steering wheel will behave erratically.

If you are driving when the ground starts to shake, pull over to the side of the road, stop the car, and set the emergency brake. If possible, avoid stopping close to overpasses, bridges, or power lines. Don't get out of the car—you will be in danger of falling down or being hit by flying objects or passing cars. Cover your head with whatever is at hand and get as low as possible in the vehicle while you ride out the quake.

If you are on a bridge or on the approach to one, in a tunnel, or on an overpass, continue driving—slowly—until you are back on straight highway or road. Then pull over and stop as above. Be mindful of other drivers who may be panicking or abandoning their vehicles. Watch for people on the roads and for debris. Remember that traffic signals may not be working.

Once the shaking has stopped, try listening to the radio to hear about road closures and potential traffic snarls. Don't drive your car immediately after a major earthquake unless absolutely necessary. Roads may be damaged and will need to be kept clear for emergency vehicles. Before starting to drive again, look around for any hazards such as downed power lines, and watch for cracks, breaks, or obstructions in the road as you drive.

If a power line falls on your car, you are at risk of being electrocuted. Stay inside the vehicle until rescue personnel can help you.

If you must abandon your car, you might want to leave your keys in the ignition and your doors unlocked in case the car needs to be moved to free up the road or prevent it from being damaged by fire. Once you are outside your car, be extremely cautious of other drivers and aware of the possible hazards around you.

Stay Safe at Work

If an earthquake strikes while you are at work, you will need to stay put until you know it's safe to go outside. You will then need to be ready to walk home or get to a safe place from your workplace. After the Tokyo transit system ceased functioning fully and roads were blocked in the 2011 Japanese quake, many office workers walked for more than 10 kilometres (6 miles) to reach their homes in the suburbs.

For your work emergency kit, you will want some supplies that allow you to be comfortable for several hours (water, food) and to be dressed appropriately for walking (sweater, sturdy shoes). Again, you will already have many of the items your need and it should not take you long to put together a small box or bag of items. See the Work Emergency Kit Supplies list on page 143.

Make a Pet Plan

Pets are important members of many families and need special consideration when it comes to emergency preparedness. Remember that pets can become frightened during an emergency and may act in uncharacteristic ways. A calm, friendly dog may become skittish and bolt in terror during an earthquake or its aftermath. A normally placid cat may scratch and bite. Get your dog on a leash and confine your cat as soon as you notice that something is happening. Make sure your dog and cat have up-to-date contact information on their tags, or an indentifying tattoo or microchip (talk to your veterinarian). The identification will help you reunite with your pet should you become separated.

Children may be particularly concerned about the well-being of a family pet. Let children know that your preparedness plan includes pets and enlist their help with assembling a pet emergency kit. See the Pet Emergency Kit Supplies list on page 144.

Make sure your kit includes a way to move your pets safely and securely, such as a leash or portable carrier (ideally a collapsible one for easy storage and transport), and familiarize your pet with the carrier in advance if it is not something you use regularly. If you need to go to an evacuation centre of some kind, remember that many will not accept pets. You might want to check with local boarding kennels and veterinarians to find out if they plan on taking pets during an emergency. You might also want to tell a friend or neighbour where you keep your pet emergency kit in case you are not home when a quake hits and it is not possible for you to return home immediately.

Review Preparations

Once you have assembled your car and work kits, and possibly a pet kit as well, look back at what you've accomplished during the four weeks of the readiness program. Does everyone in your household know what they should do during an earthquake and where they should seek shelter? Do you have the water, food, and supplies you will need to survive for seventy-two hours? Have you eliminated the hazards in your home that might cause injuries during an earthquake? Do you feel ready? If not, make a list of anything else you need to do.

Week 4 Summary

Complete your preparations with the help of these checklists found at the end of the book:

· Week 4 Checklist

· Car Emergency Kit Supplies

· Work Emergency Kit Supplies

· Pet Emergency Kit Supplies

CAN ANIMALS PREDICT EARTHQUAKES?

Many people believe that animals have the ability to detect signs of impending earthquakes, and cite ancient and more recent examples as evidence.

Reporting on the powerful earthquake and tsunami that destroyed the Greek city of Helike in 373 BC, the Roman writer Aelian wrote in *On Animals*, "For five days before [Helike] disappeared, all the mice and martens and snakes and centipedes and beetles and every other creature of that kind in the city left in a body by the road that leads to Keryneia. And the people of [Helike] seeing this happening were filled with amazement, but were unable to guess the reason. But after these creatures had departed, an earthquake occurred in the night; the city subsided; an immense wave flooded and [Helike] disappeared."

Haicheng, China, was evacuated one day before being struck by a devastating magnitude 7.6 earthquake in 1975. Many say the strange behaviour of animals—stampeding horses, caterwauling cats, snakes emerging from hibernation in the dead of winter—prompted the evacuation, although others claim that alert officials responding effectively to a series of foreshocks were responsible for saving thousands of lives.

Observers say that before the devastating Sumatra quake in 2004, the Kuwauin—a type of pheasant known for its ability to predict major earthquakes up to two days before they strike—sounded an alarm. As well, elephants and other animals moved to higher ground well before the tsunami, and a few lucky people followed them.

And in April 2009, British researchers studying the common toad in central Italy observed a mass exodus of the intuitive amphibian. Days later, a magnitude 6.3 earthquake hit the region, killing more than 150 people and causing extensive damage to the nearby town of L'Aquila.

Sixth sense or heightened senses? Some suggest that animals are able to detect pre-seismic cues such as vibrations or the release of gases and charged particles. Others claim that animals, closer to the ground and more in tune with movement in the Earth, sense the small P-wave that travels fastest from the earthquake source and arrives before the larger S-wave, which we less-sensitive humans feel. Others speculate that animals are tuned into magnetic fields variation in advance of an earthquake. But precisely what animals sense, if they feel anything at all, is a mystery.

seven

BEYOND THE ESSENTIALS
QUAKE-PROOFING AND INSURING YOUR HOME

ALTHOUGH BUILDINGS can be strengthened, there is no such thing as a completely earthquake-proof building. No one can predict exactly what will happen to any structure during a major seismic event. The magnitude and duration of the quake can lead to a wide variety of results. If your home is close to the epicentre of a major quake, structural damage is more likely, but there is no way to anticipate the exact seismic stress your home will experience. That being said, there are seismic improvements you can make that will greatly minimize the risk of damage to your home, and to the people in it. Some of these you may be able to do yourself; others will likely require the professional expertise of a builder or structural engineer. Because earthquake-proofing a structure can be expensive and time-consuming, you may want to work with a structural engineer on a five-year plan and revisit it each year.

Understand Building Codes
Most current building codes in earthquake zones around the world take seismic risks into account. It's good to

remember, though, that standard building codes address life safety; that is, they are designed to protect life rather than buildings from damage. The codes are intended to ensure the building will remain standing long enough for people to get out safely. Only buildings that house essential services and need to be up and running at all times—hospitals, police and fire stations—are built to a higher standard. Why the difference? Mostly because the higher the standard, the more expensive these buildings are to construct.

Most homes constructed in 1990 and later have seismic safety features included. For homes built before this time, consult with a structural engineer to confirm whether your home has such features, or whether upgrades or retrofits (when an already built structure is reinforced) are needed.

Secure Foundations and Chimneys

Many homes on the west coast of North America are wood-frame construction. This gives them a bit of flexibility and means that they—like the trees they are made from—can bend rather than break and thus do quite well in an earthquake. However, much damage has still occurred during major earthquakes when wood-frame houses have slid off their foundations and their inflexible brick chimneys have collapsed.

A house can be stopped from sliding by bolting it directly onto the foundation. Your house may already be bolted, something you can check by looking in your basement and garage for foundation bolts. They are placed approximately 2 metres (6 feet apart) along the sill plate and the concrete foundation. If you don't find these reassuring bolts, you might want to contact a builder. Chimneys, too, can be secured with bracing. However, this will not help all chimneys—some can be upgraded but some will need to be replaced.

The chimney on my house should be replaced. It's tall, brick, and unreinforced, and in an earthquake it would likely topple and fall through our roof and skylights into our living room. When our budget allows, we will attach a prefabricated metal chimney to the existing brick. If your chimney is in better shape than mine, you or a builder can use sheet-metal straps and angle braces to attach it to the roof and prevent it from breaking away at the roof line. This will allow you to avoid what happened in the Nisqually 2001 earthquake in Washington, where hundreds of chimneys snapped off and collapsed, causing extensive damage and injury.

Reinforce Support Walls

The vertical studs that support the floor and exterior walls of the your home—called "cripple" or "pony" walls—can buckle under severe ground motion, causing the house to collapse into its basement or crawl space. You can strengthen cripple walls by nailing plywood sheeting to the vertical studs. Again, this is something you can do yourself, but you may be more comfortable hiring a builder.

Prepare for Liquefaction

Rather than the dramatic, gaping chasms seen in disaster movies, one of the most common sights after an earthquake is a big, slimy mess. During an earthquake, shaking can cause loosely packed, water-saturated soil to turn from a solid to a liquid. This effect, known as liquefaction, can make structures lean or settle unevenly as the soil loses its strength, causing bridges to buckle and underground utility lines to rupture.

To find out if the soil that supports your home is at risk, see if a liquefaction hazard map is posted on your local government website or have a soil engineer check. If your

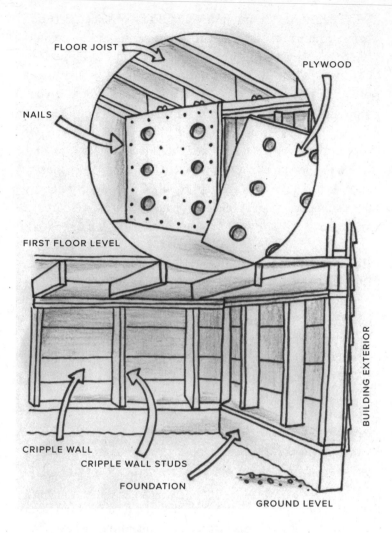

FLOOR JOIST

PLYWOOD

NAILS

FIRST FLOOR LEVEL

BUILDING EXTERIOR

CRIPPLE WALL

CRIPPLE WALL STUDS

FOUNDATION

GROUND LEVEL

Nailing plywood to the studs beneath your floor joists can strengthen the cripple walls and help them withstand the sideways movement caused by an earthquake.

home is situated on potentially unstable soil, you should reinforce your foundation and discuss other options with a structural engineer. Be happy if you learn your home is situated on dense soil or bedrock—a rock formation that extends deep into the Earth's crust. During an earthquake, the vibration travelling through your foundation will be far less and you won't have to worry about liquefaction.

Consider Earthquake Insurance

You probably have homeowner insurance—fire insurance and theft insurance, and insurance in case somebody slips on your stairs and gets hurt. You may assume that this insurance also covers any loss or damage caused by an earthquake. Well, the most important thing to know is that most homeowner insurance policies do *not* cover earthquake loss. In addition, some policies do not cover fire damage if the fire is caused by an earthquake—a very common occurrence.

Some insurers will allow you to purchase an earthquake rider (an add-on policy). Deciding whether or not to do this requires you to make some complex financial calculations involving a number of factors: your overall earthquake risk (where you live and the structural state of your home), the value of your belongings, the cost of insurance premiums, the deductible (the portion of a claim not covered by the insurer), and your overall financial situation.

Most earthquake insurance policies have a high deductible (the amount you must pay before you receive any compensation after you make a claim). This means you will be covered if your home is destroyed but perhaps not if it's merely damaged. In high-risk zones like the west coast of North America, the average deductions range from five percent to twenty percent of the value of the property. So with a deductible of ten percent, if your house is worth $400,000, the damages would need to exceed $40,000 before you could start to collect on an insurance claim.

One way to manoeuvre through the insurance minefield is to find out more about the actual costs of the damage you might face. To do this you would need to hire a structural engineer to estimate the cost of retrofitting your home and to estimate what the damage might be after an earthquake with *and* without these property-saving repairs.

At the end of your deliberations about retrofitting and potential damage, if you decide the likely cost of damage will be much higher than the insurance deductible, you might want to buy earthquake insurance. You might also decide to buy earthquake insurance if you simply want the peace of mind it brings you.

In any case, don't count on much government help after an earthquake. Homeowners, business owners, and tenants are expected to insure themselves. After an earthquake, the priority for governments will be to rebuild costly infrastructure, although there may be money for uninsurable repairs and financial assistance in the form of low-interest loans.

If you are a condo owner, your building may be covered by your strata council's insurance. This policy will, however, have a high deductible if you are in earthquake country, and your personal property will not be covered. You will need to add earthquake coverage to your own condo homeowner policy if you want to guarantee coverage. You may be able to include coverage in this for your portion of the deductible in the event that the entire building is a writeoff after a major earthquake. For example, if your entire condominium building or townhouse complex is valued at $8 million, the deductible at ten percent would be \$800,000. After the strata council reserve fund is exhausted to pay the deductible, the remainder of the cost would be divided among the condo owners. If you have a homeowner condo policy that includes earthquake coverage, some of this deductible—usually up to a maximum amount—would be covered.

If you rent your home, you should know that your landlord's insurance may not cover earthquake damage to your belongings. In the event that the ceiling of your apartment collapses on your expensive entertainment centre, it's possible that neither your landlord's building insurance nor your own tenant contents insurance will cover the damage. Again, for guaranteed coverage you would need special—and costly—earthquake insurance.

Whether you are a tenant or a homeowner, you should check with an insurance agent about the coverage you have and the coverage you may want to obtain.

A VIOLENT JOGGLING UP AND DOWN

In *Roughing It,* story-teller and humorist Mark Twain describes his youthful escapades in the American West. One adventure he recounts involves an earthquake in San Francisco in 1865.

It was just after noon, on a bright October day. I was coming down Third Street. The only objects in motion anywhere in sight in that thickly built and populous quarter were a man in a buggy behind me, and a streetcar wending slowly up the cross street. Otherwise, all was solitude and a Sabbath stillness.

As I turned the corner, around a frame house, there was a great rattle and jar, and it occurred to me that here was an item!—no doubt a fight in that house. Before I could turn and seek the door, there came a terrific shock; the ground seemed to roll under me in waves, interrupted by a violent joggling up and down, and there was a heavy grinding noise as of brick houses rubbing together ... a third and still severer shock came, and as I reeled about on the pavement trying to keep my footing, I saw a sight! The entire front of a tall four-story brick building on Third Street sprung outward like a door and fell sprawling across the street, raising a great dust-like volume of smoke!

And here came the buggy—overboard went the man, and in less time than I can tell it the vehicle was distributed in small fragments along three hundred yards of street... The streetcar had stopped, the horses were rearing and plunging, the passengers were pouring out at both ends, and one fat man had crashed halfway through a glass window on one side of the car, got wedged fast, and was squirming and screaming like an impaled madman. Every door, of every house, as far as the eye could reach, was vomiting a stream of human beings; and almost before one could execute a wink and begin another, there was a massed multitude of people stretching in endless procession down every street my position commanded. Never was a solemn solitude turned into teeming life quicker.

eight

DURING AN
EARTHQUAKE

YOU WILL likely hear the rumbling first. Or perhaps experience a jolt. The rumbling may build to a deafening roar
sounding like thunder or a high-speed train. The ground
will begin to shake and roll violently, maybe for several
seconds or perhaps for what feels like an eternity—several
minutes. The longer the shaking, the greater the damage.
This is where all your psychological preparation will pay off.
You've become earthquake aware and although you will
be terrified when you first feel the ground move, you will
know what to do.

Put Your Plan into Action

This is the time to lead. Remind yourself and others to act
as planned and to take the essential steps summarized in
What to Do When the Ground Shakes on page 145. Give
loud, clear directions—to yourself if you are alone or to
others who are present—"Drop, cover, and hold on!" Take
shelter under a desk, table, or bench and hold onto a table
leg or other sturdy object. Keep talking yourself and others
through the experience. Minimize your movements.

If You Are Indoors

- Stay indoors until the shaking stops. Remember most injuries during an earthquake occur when people enter or exit buildings.

- If you are in a place you do not know well, quickly scan the room for hazards you might need to avoid—windows, light fixtures, tall furniture.

- If there isn't a table or desk near you, grab what you can find to protect your head and neck—pillows, coats, magazines—or cover your head and neck with your arms and crouch in an inside corner of the building with your back against the wall.

- If you are in a crowded room, do not run to the exit. Stay in the centre of the room, away from windows, and drop, cover, and hold on.

- If you are in bed, stay there. Pull up the covers and grab a pillow. Wait for the shaking to stop.

- If you are in the kitchen, turn off the stove. Move to a safe place. If this is a kitchen you do not know well, get away from cupboards and appliances. Protect your head as you move to safety.

- Wherever you are indoors, do not stand in a doorway *unless* this has been previously identified as a safe place: a strong load-bearing doorframe without a door to swing shut in a place unlikely to be used as an exit point by people trying to leave the building.

If You Are Outdoors

- Again, minimize your movement until the shaking stops.

- If you are in an open field, stay there. Just look out for trees and power lines and crouch down with your head covered.

- If you are near tall buildings, move into the doorway overhang of a building or a lobby to protect yourself from falling masonry and glass.

- If you are on a street or sidewalk, move away from building walls, chimneys, streetlights, and utility poles. Couch down and cover your head.

If You Are in Other Locations

- If you are in a theatre or stadium, do not leave your seat. Cover you head and wait until the shaking stops.

- If you are in an airplane, consider yourself lucky for you will not feel the effects of an earthquake. You may, however, have some difficulty landing and need to be re-routed if there is serious damage at your destination.

- If you are in a parking garage in your car, stop the car, get under the dashboard and tell others to get as low as possible in the vehicle.

- If you are on a beach, look for cover close by and move to higher ground as soon as the shaking stops in case a tsunami is coming. (See Chapter 9 for more details about tsunamis.)

Tips for Children

Because of their smaller size, children are particularly vulnerable to injury from falling or flying objects. If my flat-screen TV landed on top of me, I might not be hurt. A small child could be seriously injured.

Practising drop, cover, and hold on with children is particularly important, since they will naturally be tempted to run through the house looking for other family members and pets. Use every opportunity to reinforce the importance of staying put until the shaking of an earthquake stops.

THE TRIANGLE OF LIFE: A MISGUIDED
IDEA ABOUT EARTHQUAKE SAFETY

Several years ago, an earthquake safety method was circulated widely and embraced by many. This method, called the Triangle of Life, was spread through email and social media, and pinned to countless bulletin boards. Today, all official and reliable sources of earthquake safety information reject this "misguided idea," as the U.S. Geological Survey calls it, and continue to recommend that you drop, cover, and hold on.

In short, the proponents of the Triangle of Life maintain that if you are in a house or other building when an earthquake strikes, the safest place to be is *beside* a piece of furniture rather than *underneath* a table or desk. This is based on the idea that any large pieces of structural debris—ceiling beams, for example— will hit the surface of the furniture, and form an empty "triangle" of space in which you will be safe.

The idea makes some theoretical sense, especially when applied to developing countries where structural collapse is common. However, as any credible earthquake safety source will tell you, there is no predicting where structural debris will fall or settle, and this kind of hazard is the least of your worries. In developed parts of the world, most earthquake deaths and injuries are caused by the household items and building materials—dishes, books, bricks, and glass shards—that become high-speed projectiles. The worst thing you can do is to run around looking for a "safer" place where a triangle *might* form *if* a large structural component falls. The movement of the quake is likely to toss you around as you run, and your exposed body will be a target for objects flying from all directions.

The absolute best thing you can do is drop, cover, and hold on.

nine

AFTER AN
EARTHQUAKE

IN THE moments after an earthquake you may find yourself in darkness. You may be covered in dust and papers,
books, or glass. You may be wet from sprinklers going off
in the office where you were working moments before. The
urge to get outside as quickly as possible will be more than
intense—it will be instinctual and most likely a wrong and
dangerous urge to give in to.

In the moments following an earthquake you are likely
to find yourself in a state of hyper-awareness—extremely
awake and focused on survival. However, know that reactions will vary even among those who are in the same
location when the quake hits. In the 9.0 megathrust earthquake in Japan in 2011, people's reactions varied depending
upon where they were. Office workers stranded on the
thirty-fifth floor of a Tokyo tower feared for their lives,
while in a nearby park a group of boys continued to play
soccer, seemingly oblivious of the people streaming past.

This is when preparation and practice will help you do
the right thing, the safest thing, rather than the thing that
comes to mind first. Now is the time to use the information you have recorded in your emergency communication

plan and the supplies you have organized in your home emergency kit, car emergency kit, work emergency kit, or personal grab-and-go bag. Now is also the time for household members, including children, to do the jobs they have been assigned and that you have planned for and practised. For example, you may have delegated a teen to be in charge of turning off the electricity, an older child to get the home emergency kit, and a younger child to take care of pets while you send a text message to your non-local emergency contact.

If you find yourself trapped under debris (or need to advise a trapped family member, neighbour, or co-worker), remember the following:

- Do not move quickly or try to shout, since you may stir up and inhale dangerous amounts of dust or other fine debris.

- If you are able to move, the first thing you should do is to cover your mouth—use a handkerchief or part of your clothing.

- Keep yourself calm by counting your breaths.

- Tap on a pipe or wall or whatever is close and solid so that rescuers can find you.

Check for Injuries, Damage, and Hazards
Once you are able to stand and move around after an earthquake, check yourself and others for injuries. Unless someone has an immediately life-threatening injury, look after your own injuries first so that you are able to help others. Refer to the first aid manual in your home emergency kit if necessary.

Check for structural damage. Look for deep surface cracks, broken studs, or stucco damage. Do not enter an unstable building for any reason. You risk disrupting a delicate balance and causing more damage or injury.

Check for hazards such as gas leaks, ruptured water lines, exposed electrical wires, and fires.

Deal with Gas, Water, and Electricity

An earthquake can do significant damage to gas lines, water lines, and electrical systems, both outside and inside your home. This can lead to fires, flooded basements, and power surges. One of your first jobs once the shaking stops will be to check on your home's utility services and, if necessary, turn off the gas, electricity, and water.

Turning Off Gas

If your house is heated by natural gas, or if you have a gas stove, an earthquake could crack or rupture the pipes that carry the gas into your home. A leak can be extremely dangerous as the flowing gas may be ignited by the smallest spark and cause an explosion. Gas companies add a substance to natural gas so that it's easy to detect a leak. A sour, sulfur odour (like rotten eggs) indicates that you have a gas leak. Depending on the source of the leak, you may also hear a hissing sound.

If you do not smell gas or hear a hissing sound, do *not* turn off your gas. You won't be able to turn it back on by yourself—only a qualified gas fitter can restore the gas supply. After an earthquake this could take days or weeks and would present a problem during cold weather when you need gas for heating and cooking.

If you *do* smell gas or hear hissing and suspect a gas leak, turn off the gas at once. To do this, you will need to use a wrench and turn the valve on the meter one-quarter turn to either the left or right.

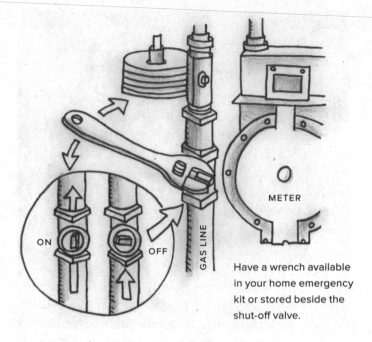

METER

ON

OFF

GAS LINE

Have a wrench available in your home emergency kit or stored beside the shut-off valve.

As well as turning off the gas when you suspect a leak, it is very important to do the following:

- Do not turn electrical switches on or off.

- Do not light matches or use lighters.

- Extinguish any cigarettes, candles, and other open flames.

- Leave a door or window open.

- Exit the building immediately.

- Notify the gas company if possible.

Turning Off Water

Even without an earthquake, water pipes can burst for a number of reasons, including corrosion, freezing

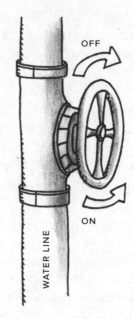

Label your water line or paint an arrow nearby to help anyone looking for the shut-off valve.

OFF

ON

WATER LINE

temperatures, and accidents. Broken water pipes can quickly lead to a contaminated water supply and property damage. Every person in your home should know how to shut down the supply. There are two shut-off valves, one inside and one outside. Your priority is the inside one.

> **Inside water shut-off valve.** This is usually in the basement or on the main floor. I lived in one house where it was on the basement ceiling, covered up by a ceiling tile. Make sure everyone knows where your water valve is located. To shut off the water, turn the valve all the way to the right.

> **Outside water shut-off valve.** You will also probably have an outside shut-off valve. Usually this will be under a circular cover at the front of the house or apartment building, near

the road or on the lawn. This valve is trickier to turn off as it often requires a special water key that you must obtain from a plumber, your local fire service, or another municipal authority.

Turning Off Electricity

A major earthquake will likely disrupt power in many areas. If the power is off in your neighbourhood, house, or apartment building, shutting off your electricity will help protect against power surges that could do further damage to your electrical system (and to any items that are plugged in at the time). Shutting off electricity is also a good idea if you need to evacuate. It may prevent fire if the power comes back on when you're not home. Make sure everyone in your household knows the location of your electrical box, and understands how to switch off the main power supply.

Control Fires

Fires often follow close on the heels of an earthquake. Fire after a seismic event can be the result of broken gas lines, overturned heaters, and severed electrical connections. The situation can be made worse when water mains are damaged and fire-fighting teams are unable to get past fallen trees and power lines. You can expect earthquake damage and fires to keep your local fire fighters busy, and should therefore be prepared to deal with fire if it breaks out in your home, office, or car.

Keep two small extinguishers rather than a single large one. Place them in different rooms and—if your home has more than one storey—on different floors.

Look for a Class ABC type of extinguisher, which is capable of putting out fires involving paper, wood, and most other combustibles (A), flammable liquids such as gasoline, paint remover, and grease (B), and electrical fires (C).

It may seem straightforward, but it's important to read the instructions that come with your fire extinguisher. Go through the motions of pretending to put out a fire. Better yet, take some training from your local fire department. Haven't you always wanted to let loose with a fire extinguisher?

PASS is a mnemonic that will help you use an extinguisher properly. It reminds you to:

- **P**ull the pin found at the top of the extinguisher to release the locking mechanism.

- **A**im the nozzle at the base of the fire to target the fuel that feeds the fire.

- **S**queeze the trigger slowly while holding the extinguisher upright.

- **S**weep from side to side covering the area of the fire.

You may want to take the card containing this information (page 146) and put it near your fire extinguisher or tape it right onto the cartridge. Be aware that the most common fires after an earthquake are electrical fires and those fueled by gas or oil and grease. You should never use water on any of these kinds of fire. Use a fire extinguisher, and in the case of an electrical or gas fire, turn off the electricity as soon as possible. Throw baking soda on a grease fire if you can.

Of course there are times when you should not try to fight a fire and should evacuate immediately:

- If the fire is spreading rapidly.

- If the fire may soon block your escape route.

The most important thing is to be able to get out of the building and away from the fire and smoke. Once you're out, stay out. Under no circumstances should you enter a smoke-filled building. Smoke contains toxic chemicals and hot gases than can quickly cause serious and permanent damage.

Take the Next Steps

Once you have addressed any life- or property-threatening emergencies, you can proceed with other tasks. Begin by making sure your telephone is working. After you've called your non-local contact, avoid making other unnecessary calls so that phone lines will be free for the use of emergency responders.

Turn on your windup or battery-powered radio. This will be your most reliable source for news of what's happening locally and other essential information. If damage is severe, reliable information may be scarce for several days following the quake.

Take a deep breath and get ready for some clean-up. Be careful entering rooms and opening cupboards and closets in the same way you are when retrieving items from overhead bins on an airplane after a flight—objects may have shifted during the recent turbulence.

Cleaning Up

Clearing away debris and assessing damage will occupy a good portion of your time immediately after a quake. If possible, take photos of your home and belongings, from different angles and distances, before you begin to clean up. If you can't take photos, start a list and make sketches of what you find. A good record of the damage will make filing an insurance claim easier later.

Carefully begin to clean up debris, watching for broken glass and damaged electrical cords. Make sure the power is switched off before touching anything electrical to avoid being electrocuted. Once you turn the power back on, check your appliances for damage, especially if there was a power outage and an electrical surge.

If water lines broke anywhere in your home, look for water damage and do what you can to mop up and dry out your belongings.

Managing Food and Water

As you clean up your kitchen and take stock of supplies, be aware that shattered glass may have fallen into any open containers of food. In the days immediately after an earthquake, plan meals that use the perishable food in your refrigerator and freezer first; you can use the longer-lasting canned and dried food on your kitchen shelves and in your home emergency kit later. Even without electricity, and depending on what you have stored, your chilled and frozen food should remain usable for two to three days if you keep the refrigerator and freezer doors closed.

Listen to the radio for water safety advisories. If your water is unsafe or has been turned off, use the water in your home emergency kit. If this runs out, turn to alternative sources, as mentioned in Chapter 3: melted ice cubes, the liquid from canned fruit and vegetables, water from your hot water tank, and water from your toilet tank with bleach added.

Expecting the Best

Despite what we see in media reports that focus on looting, violence, and other forms of bad behaviour after a disaster, studies show that the vast majority of people behave responsibly and even nobly. The admirable civility of the Japanese under the dire circumstances of the 2011 earthquake, tsunami, and nuclear power plant failure supports this. "When the crunch comes, and the world begins to fall apart, the true, raw self comes out—and we find it's essentially humane," says Kathleen Tierney, director of the Disaster Research Center at the University of Delaware. "The point," Tierney says, "is that altruism is not all that exceptional; it's the rule."

During an emergency, try to expect the best from people, and—as much as possible—become the best, most helpful and compassionate person you can be. Rather than giving in to fear and panic, go check on your neighbours.

Evacuate if Necessary

After an earthquake, you may need to evacuate if your home is not safe structurally, if you need medical attention, or if an official evacuation order is made for your area. Otherwise, it is best to stay in your home even if your power is out, your water is off, and your house is a mess of broken objects. The emergency shelters will be there if you need them, but they will be overcrowded and will, at least initially, lack basic services. Your ability to take care of yourself for at least the first seventy-two hours after an earthquake will allow service providers to tend to the most critical emergencies.

If you do have to evacuate, take comfort from the fact that most local and regional governments in North America have sophisticated emergency response plans. The province of B.C., for example, has a disaster response route program designed to prevent the traffic chaos that has happened after many disasters. These networks of designated roads, rail, water, and air routes will be used to move emergency service providers and supplies as quickly as possible to the areas most in need. The province also has a reception centre program that will see schools and other public facilities open up to receive people stranded or hurt. In the mean-time, search-and-rescue teams will look for survivors and emergency social service and communication teams will begin to offer support.

Watch for Aftershocks

Earthquakes usually happen in clusters, with foreshocks, the main shock, and aftershocks. The earthquake with the largest magnitude is the main shock; anything that occurs before it is a foreshock and anything after is an aftershock.

Aftershocks occur as the Earth's crust resettles and the stress caused by the main quake is redistributed along the fault line. Most aftershocks will occur close in location and time to the main shock, but they can also continue for days, months, and even years after. Although individual earthquakes are unpredictable, aftershocks follow known patterns. Not surprisingly, the bigger the earthquake, the bigger the aftershock.

It's important to remember that any large earthquake will be followed by a number of aftershocks within the first hour or two. Aftershocks can be as dangerous as the main earthquake since they can complete the damage started by the main shock—damaged buildings may tumble to the ground, and roads or bridges that apparently survived the main shock may crumble. The same rule that applies to earthquakes applies to aftershocks—drop, cover, and hold on.

Watch for Tsunamis

Tsunami is a Japanese word made up of two characters: *tsu*, meaning "harbour" and *nami*, meaning "wave." Many people refer to tsunamis as tidal waves, but this is a misno-mer, since tsunamis are not connected to the natural cycle of tides. Rather, a tsunami is a series of long ocean waves caused by an extreme and sudden disturbance of the ocean floor. These long waves can travel for many thousands of kilometres at the speed of a jet—more than 700 kilometres (435 miles) per hour—before slamming into land. The scale of devastation caused by tsunamis makes them particularly frightening. The 2004 Sumatra earthquake triggered a series of deadly tsunamis that claimed thousands of lives in fourteen different countries.

Although tsunamis can be deadly, not all earthquakes cause tsunamis. For a tsunami to be generated there must be vertical movement on the ocean floor, which of course means the earthquake's epicentre must be close to or under an ocean. If you live far inland (and have no plans for an oceanside holiday) you can scratch tsunamis off your worry list. But if you live on the coast, you need to be aware of how tsunamis operate and how to prepare for them.

Tsunamis are caused by earthquakes but they can also be generated by landslides, volcanic eruptions, and even on rare occasions by falling meteorites. Earthquake-generated tsunamis happen at subduction zones—those dangerous sites on the Earth's crust where drifting plates converge. Remember that when these enormous plates give way, the release of pressure can result in an earthquake that lifts and shifts thousands of square kilometres of the Earth—in this case, the floor of the ocean. The energy from this explosive movement along the fault is transferred to the ocean above, displacing enormous volumes of water, propelling it upward, and causing a wave to form.

Normally, the size and power of ocean waves are determined by the strength of the wind and tides. In the case of a tsunami, the size and power are determined by the magnitude of the earthquake. Wind-generated waves can reach

heights of 30 metres (100 feet) or more—these are the curl-
ing waves surfers adore. The highest recorded tsunami was
more than twice that size—85 metres (278 feet)—off the
coast of Ryukyu Island in Japan in 1971.

As the tsunami reaches the coastline, its speed dimin-
ishes while its height increases—a result of the mass of
water meeting the shallow ocean floor. The waves become
compressed like an accordion while the energy in this
smaller volume of water begins to concentrate in a process called shoaling. We witnessed the destructive power
of shoaling when boats—including very large ones—were
lifted in the bays and harbours of northeastern Japan in
2011 and hurled violently against the shore. The waves of a
tsunami can travel 2 kilometres or more inland, flattening
buildings and displacing anything in their path. Tsunamis
can also travel up rivers and streams that lead to the ocean.

The destruction caused by a tsunami is less about the
height of the wave and more about the length and the large
volume of water that pours on to the shoreline. Often a
tsunami won't break like a normal wave when it reaches
the shore, which makes it look deceptively smaller than
it really is. The force of some tsunamis is enormous. Large
rocks weighing several tonnes can be moved inland hundreds of metres by a tsunami wave.

Warning Systems

It's important to know that the first sign of a tsunami can
be water receding quickly and to a significant distance.
Fortunately, those living in areas at risk may receive an
even earlier sign through tsunami alert centres. Tsunami
warning systems have been set up in coastal areas around
the world. Not surprisingly, most are found on the Pacific
Ring of Fire, with Japan's being the most advanced system

in the world. The system detects tremors from seismic monitoring stations, calculates an earthquake's epicentre, and sends out warnings within seconds of the first waves of an earthquake.

When the magnitude 9.0 earthquake struck off Japan's northeast coast in 2011, it took mere seconds for a seismometer near the epicentre to detect enough P-wave signals to determine that an earthquake alert was necessary. The alert was automatically issued to schools, factories, news networks, and to mobile phones. The more damaging but later-arriving S-waves reached Tokyo—370 kilometres (230 miles) to the south—in ninety seconds, enough time for many to take cover, pull over, or stop machinery. Within nine minutes of the quake, a tsunami warning was also issued. This allowed about fifteen minutes for those in the hardest-hit areas to respond. We know the devastation and loss of life that ensued, but contrast this with Japan's deadliest earthquake—the Kanto earthquake of 1923 (with a magnitude of 7.9)—which killed between 120,000 and 150,000 people. In 2011 the warning system worked, the Japanese were prepared, and the country responded as well as circumstances allowed. Thousands of lives were saved.

Before
All low-lying coastal areas can be struck by tsunamis. Vulnerable areas include beaches on the open ocean, entrances to bays and harbours, tidal flats, and the shore along coastal rivers and inlets with exposure to the open ocean.

If you live in or are heading to a vulnerable area, assess the risks and make sure you have an evacuation plan in place beforehand—including a plan to leave your home, your school, your workplace, your picnic spot, or camping site. Check a hazard map to find out which areas are most at risk during a tsunami. Watch for warning signs posted in areas that might be inundated and signs indicating that you are on a tsunami evacuation route. When you are at a beach or in a tsunami hazard zone, maintain your situational awareness by taking note of any routes to higher ground. Discuss these locations with your loved ones, particularly your children.

During and After

If you hear a warning for a tsunami generated by an earthquake thousands of kilometres away, get your grab-and-go bag and head for higher ground. Do not wait until you can see the tsunami approaching. And do not wait to watch the waves strike the shore. It's almost impossible to outrun a tsunami so every second counts. Remember that tsunamis generally involve several powerful waves, so do not return to the shore if you see the water start to recede. Many people have died when the second wave of a tsunami hits.

If you are near the ocean or at the beach and you feel an earthquake, drop, cover, and hold on, as you would anytime the ground shakes. As soon as the shaking stops, immediately move inland or to higher ground. Do not wait for an official warning. If you are camping or picnicking, be prepared to abandon your belongings. Your life could be in danger.

If you are on a boat in deep ocean water, the tsunami may pass unnoticed under you. If you are on a boat in a harbour when a tsunami is approaching, you will have to decide whether or not you have time to get to shore and higher ground, or if you should try to leave the harbour for open water. What you do will depend on the size of your boat and your exact location. In any case, be aware of your surroundings and conscious of the tsunami warning systems and communication plans in your location. Stay in contact with the local port authority and listen to their advice.

After a tsunami, wait for emergency response officials to give the "all clear" before you return to your home, boat, or car. Be aware that driving could be extremely dangerous and watch for hazardous debris and damaged roads and bridges.

Recovery

Once the debris from a major earthquake or other disaster has been cleared and your situation is returning to normal, you may be surprised to find yourself still affected by your experiences. You may feel that the world has changed, and all aspects of your life—your emotions, your thoughts, and even your values—have shifted. These changes can be both challenging and positive.

On the positive side, the intensity of experiencing and surviving an emergency can increase your appreciation for friends, family, neighbours, and life in general. The usual day-to-day worries vanish for a time as you are forced to focus on the present. Your sense of what is most important in life can come into sharp focus.

Some of the more challenging—and very normal—reactions can be continued fear followed by shock and numbness, as well as a sense of frustration, anger, helplessness, and a lot of grief and despair. It may all seem like too much to bear. Remember that you have just been through a traumatic event. It will likely take time before you start to feel normal.

Work on discovering some positive ways to cope, such as getting involved in efforts to provide comfort and support to others in your family and community. Stay busy and get involved in practical tasks. Make sure you and your family members get nutritious food, plenty of rest, and sufficient exercise. Re-establish routines and limit your exposure to news accounts of the disaster on TV, the radio, online, and in newspapers.

Give yourself time to recover, but don't be afraid to ask for help if you're not sleeping, or if you notice that you're always on edge, agitated, or irritable. If you're feeling numb or hopeless, or if you're having recurrent nightmares or thinking about your experiences nonstop, then it's time to seek professional help.

Children often experience more anxiety than adults after a disaster because they feel their entire world is out of control. Some children will need a lot of reassurance and should be reminded to use the breathing techniques described in Chapter 2. Hug your children often, and tell them they are safe. Remember that a child who has been prepared for a crisis and who has experienced wise leadership by prepared adults will feel safer both during and after.

As you move through the days following an earthquake or other disaster, help yourself and your family with the following strategies:

> **Communicate.** Talk about what has happened and is happening. Make opportunities for communication in your family rather than leaving it to chance.

> **Share information.** Let your children know what's going on. Reality is easier to deal with than fear of the unknown.

> **Have fun.** Take a break from the clean-up and recovery tasks to play.

> **Keep family roles clear.** Don't allow children to take on too much responsibility. You don't want to overprotect them

but you don't want to leave them without adult care and support either.

> **Be active and involved.** Help others tackle problems and seek the help you need yourself.

> **Take time to reflect on what you've learned.** Share your story with others inside and outside the family.

> **Be patient.** After a disaster, some people will be more distressed than others. Allow yourself and others time to heal.

A NOBLE EARTHQUAKE

Beloved nature writer and conservationist John Muir describes the great Owens Valley earthquake of 1872 in his book *The Yosemite.*

At half-past two o'clock of a moonlit morning in March, I was awakened by a tremendous earthquake, and though I had never before enjoyed a storm of this sort, the strange thrilling motion could not be mistaken, and I ran out of my cabin, both glad and frightened, shouting, "A noble earthquake! A noble earthquake!" feeling sure I was going to learn something.

The shocks were so violent and varied, and succeeded one another so closely, that I had to balance myself carefully in walking as if on the deck of a ship among waves, and it seemed impossible that the high cliffs of the Valley could escape being shattered. In particular, I feared that the sheer-fronted Sentinel Rock, towering above my cabin, would be shaken down, and I took shelter back of a large yellow pine, hoping that it might protect me from at least the smaller outbounding boulders.

For a minute or two the shocks became more and more violent— flashing horizontal thrusts mixed with a few twists and battering, explosive, upheaving jolts—as if Nature were wrecking her Yosemite

*temple, and getting ready to build a still better one…No sound was
heard for the first minute or so [after the earthquake], save low, muffled,
underground, bubbling rumblings, and the whispering and rustling of
the agitated trees, as if Nature were holding her breath. Then, suddenly,
out of the strange silence and strange motion there came a tremendous
roar. The Eagle Rock on the south wall, about a half a mile up the Valley, gave way and I saw it falling in thousands of the great boulders I
had so long been studying, pouring to the Valley floor in a free curve
luminous from friction, making a terribly sublime spectacle—an arc of
glowing, passionate fire, fifteen hundred feet span, as true in form and
as serene in beauty as a rainbow in the midst of the stupendous, roar-
ing rockstorm.*

*After the ground began to calm I ran across the meadow to the river
to see in what direction it was flowing and was glad to find that* down
the Valley was still down.

CONCLUSION

I STILL experience moments of doubt, especially when I look at a book or website that terrifies me with worst-case scenarios. After I'm briefly stricken by fear and fatalism, I remind myself that I have hugely increased my chances of surviving an earthquake by having some supplies on hand and a plan in place. To reinforce my commitment to getting ready, I revisit one of my supplies lists, check my calendar for the family preparedness day we've scheduled for the switch to daylight savings time, and look at the expiry date on my kitchen fire extinguisher. I encourage you to do the same and not get derailed by doubt.

If you have completed the readiness program described here, you will now have:

- Developed an emergency communication plan.

- Eliminated many hazards from your home.

- Practised drop, cover, and hold on.

- Assembled a home emergency kit and personal grab-and-go bag.

- Set dates to review your plans and refresh your supplies.

You may also have assembled emergency kits for your car, your work, and your pets. And you may have secured the foundation of your house and decided to invest in earthquake insurance.

Along the way you may have engaged your family, friends, co-workers, and neighbours in the process. Perhaps you've considered starting up a community emergency preparedness group—a fun and satisfying way to get to know your neighbours and a great way to build skills you can draw on throughout life. Maybe you've even found yourself noticing possible exits at the supermarket and practising calm breathing while waiting for the traffic lights to change. If you have children, you may have found that conversations about scary events have opened the door to other potentially scary subjects—teenage parties or plans for university.

Congratulations! You can now move through your life with a greater sense of ease, knowing that if you feel the ground shake, you will know what to do. Being prepared means you no longer have to avoid thinking and talking about what to do, nor do you have to become anxious when you see reports of disasters in different parts of the world. You can marvel at the awesome power of earthquakes, storms, and floods, while knowing that you have done what you can to look after yourself and your loved ones.

One final piece of advice: make sure you keep your dates with yourself and your household members to review plans, update information, and refresh supplies. Preparing will already have made you feel so much better about the prospect of a disaster; maintaining your preparations ensures you continue to feel this way—one of the biggest rewards of getting ready.

CHECKLISTS AND FORMS

Visit www.dmpibooks.com/event/285
to print copies.

Week 1 Checklist

☐ Enter a date in your calendar to meet with
the members of your household.

☐ Meet and develop your emergency communication plan.

☐ Determine your non-local emergency contacts.

☐ Identify your emergency reunion site.

☐ Complete a contact card for every person in your
household.

☐ Make a printed copy of your important phone numbers
for every person in your household.

☐ Go to the grocery store with the Shopping List for
Home Emergency Kit and buy any food needed.

☐ Start assembling the contents of your
home emergency kit:

    ☐ Store water.

    ☐ Store food.

☐ Enter a date in your calendar to change the water and
food in your kit in six months.

☐ Enter a date in your calendar to review your
emergency plans in twelve months.

OTHER TASKS _____

_____

Emergency Communication Plan

GIVE A COPY TO:

☐ Every member of your family or household

☐ All of your non-local emergency contacts

PUT A COPY IN YOUR:

☐ Home emergency kit

☐ Grab-and-go bags

☐ Work emergency kit

☐ Car emergency kit

NON-LOCAL EMERGENCY CONTACTS

PRIMARY CONTACT

Contact Name: _____

Home phone number: _____

Cell phone number: _____

Work phone number: _____

Email address 1: _____

Email address 2: _____

Notes: _____

SECONDARY CONTACT

Contact name: _____

Home phone number: _____

Cell phone number: _____

Work phone number: _____

Email address 1: _____

Email address 2: _____

Notes: _____

REUNION SITES

Primary reunion site

_____

_____

_____

_____

_____

_____

Alternate reunion site (if Primary is not accessible)

_____

_____

_____

_____

_____

Second alternate reunion site
(if Primary and Alternate are not accessible)

_____

_____

_____

_____

_____

If I leave home, I will leave a note in the following
location(s):

_____

_____

_____

_____

_____

_____

Contact Card

As soon as possible after an earthquake, phone your contact or have someone else call to say how you are, where you are, and what your plans are.

SIDE 1

NON-LOCAL EMERGENCY CONTACTS

PRIMARY CONTACT

Home phone: _____

Cell phone: _____

Work phone: _____

Email 1: _____

Email 2: _____

Notes: _____

SECONDARY CONTACT

Home phone: _____

Cell phone: _____

Work phone: _____

Email 1: _____

Email 2: _____

SIDE 2

REUNION SITES

PRIMARY REUNION SITE: _____
_____

ALTERNATE REUNION SITE: _____
(if Primary is not accessible)
_____

SECOND ALTERNATE REUNION SITE: _____
(if Primary and Alternate are not accessible)
_____

Shopping List for Home Emergency Kit

☐ Ready-to-eat canned vegetables, fruits, and meats

☐ Canned juice

☐ Canned milk—evaporated

☐ Canned soup

☐ Dehydrated soups and stews
(remember to store extra water for these)

☐ Dry milk and powdered drink mixes
(remember to store extra water for these)

☐ Sugar, salt, pepper, spices

☐ High-energy food—peanut butter, jam,
crackers, granola bars, trail mix bars

☐ Comfort food—cookies, coffee (instant or ground),
tea bags, hard candy (avoid sticky candies or gum—
these can melt and get into everything)

☐ Ready-to-eat cereals and granola

☐ Instant oatmeal

☐ Instant pudding

☐ Food for any household members on special
diets, such as babies, the elderly, and those with
diabetes or allergies

☐ Food for pets

NOTE: Look at the expiry date on everything you buy, keeping in mind
that you may not be eating any of those foods for the next six months.

OTHER ITEMS _____

_____

Week 2 Checklist

☐ Meet with members of your household to walk through your home and look for hazards.

☐ Use the Earthquake Hazard Hunt form to list each hazard and note how you have eliminated it or plan to eliminate it.

☐ Make sure household members know how to drop, cover, and hold on.

☐ Review the Home Emergency Kit Supplies list to determine which items you already have.

☐ Shop for any items you need.

☐ Complete your home emergency kit:

    ☐ Store cooking and eating utensils.

    ☐ Store first aid supplies.

    ☐ Store tools and other gear.

OTHER TASKS _____

_____

_____

_____

_____

_____

_____

Earthquake Hazard Hunt

Look for hazards in each room of your home:

- Heavy or fragile objects on high shelves
- Wall-mounted pictures, TV sets, mirrors, or clocks
- Hanging lights, plants, or other heavy objects
- Rolling carts holding a TV or other heavy object
- Beds placed under or beside a large window
- Electronic equipment or small appliances on high open shelves, desktops, or countertops
- Open shelf units
- Bookshelves, tall appliances, and heavy furniture
- Cabinets and cupboards with doors that might fly open
- Gas stove with an inflexible feed line
- Unsecured hot water tank

ROOM 1: _____

Item: _____

Hazard: _____

Secured: _____

Item: _____

Hazard: _____

Secured: _____

ROOM 2: _____

Item: _____

Hazard: _____

Secured: _____

Item: _____

Hazard: _____

Secured: _____

ROOM 3: _____

Item: _____

Hazard: _____

Secured: _____

Item: _____

Hazard: _____

Secured: _____

ROOM 4: _____

Item: _____

Hazard: _____

Secured: _____

Item: _____

Hazard: _____

Secured: _____

ROOM 5: _____

Item: _____

Hazard: _____

Secured: _____

Item: _____

Hazard: _____

Secured: _____

ROOM 6:_____

Item: _____

Hazard: _____

Secured: _____

Item: _____

Hazard: _____

Secured: _____

MATERIALS NEEDED TO SECURE ITEMS

_____

_____

_____

_____

_____

_____

_____

_____

Home Emergency Kit Supplies

☐ Cooking and eating utensils

☐ Can opener

☐ Aluminum foil

☐ Resealable plastic bags (small, medium, and large) for storing food and other items

☐ Unscented liquid household chlorine bleach (for purifying water and general cleaning)

☐ First aid kit, including the following:

   ☐ hydrogen peroxide

   ☐ bandages

   ☐ sterile gauze pads

   ☐ tape

   ☐ scissors

   ☐ tweezers

   ☐ antibiotic ointment

   ☐ over-the-counter pain medication

   ☐ up-to-date, comprehensive first aid manual

☐ Hand sanitizer and moist towelettes

☐ Toilet paper or tissues

☐ Lighter and matches in a waterproof container

☐ Candles

☐ Pen/pencil and paper

☐ Windup or battery-powered flashlight (and extra batteries)

- [ ] Windup or battery-powered radio (and extra batteries)
- [ ] Work gloves
- [ ] Whistle
- [ ] Heavy-duty garbage bags
- [ ] Duct tape
- [ ] Fire extinguisher
- [ ] Wrench for turning off gas
- [ ] Pocket knife (a multifunction type is best)
- [ ] Small fuel-operated stove
- [ ] Supply of fuel, ideally in small, portable canisters
- [ ] Tent or tents and tarps to shelter all household members
- [ ] Sleeping bags

OTHER ITEMS _____

_____

_____

_____

_____

_____

_____

_____

Week 3 Checklist

- [ ] Practise drop, cover, and hold with members of your household.

- [ ] Walk through your home with household members and look for safe places to shelter.

- [ ] As you go about your daily activities, look for safe places at other locations: the library, the theatre, the park, etc.

- [ ] Review the Personal Grab-and-Go Bag Supplies list to determine which items you already have.

- [ ] Shop for any items needed, including additional prescription drugs.

- [ ] Make copies of the identification cards and documents needed for each household member's personal grab-and-go bag.

- [ ] Visit a bank and withdraw cash in small-denomination bills and coins for each personal grab-and-go bag.

- [ ] Assemble personal grab-and-go bags.

OTHER TASKS _____

_____

_____

_____

_____

_____

_____

Personal Grab-and-Go Bag Supplies

- [ ] Copies of identification, including:
    - [ ] driver's licence
    - [ ] health care card
    - [ ] passport
- [ ] Copies of important documents, including:
    - [ ] contact card (information about non-local emergency contacts completed in week 1)
    - [ ] list of phone numbers
    - [ ] home insurance
    - [ ] recent bank statements
    - [ ] medical records
- [ ] Spare car keys
- [ ] Cash—small-denomination bills and coins
- [ ] T-shirt
- [ ] Sweatshirt
- [ ] Sweater
- [ ] Flat, comfortable walking shoes
- [ ] Waterproof jacket
- [ ] Comfortable pants
- [ ] Underwear and socks (three pairs of each)
- [ ] Light hat
- [ ] Mittens and toque
- [ ] Nonperishable snack such as granola bars or dried fruit

- [ ] Water—at least 1 litre (1 quart)
- [ ] Pocket knife (a multifunction type is best)
- [ ] Can opener
- [ ] Spare eye glasses and/or contact lenses and solution
- [ ] Prescription medication (enough of all medications taken for at least one week)
- [ ] Toiletry kit, including:
  - [ ] toothbrush and toothpaste
  - [ ] face cloth and towel
  - [ ] soap and shampoo
  - [ ] deodorant
  - [ ] body lotion
  - [ ] razor
  - [ ] comb or brush
  - [ ] lip balm
  - [ ] feminine hygiene products
  - [ ] vitamins
- [ ] Small first aid kit, including:
  - [ ] hydrogen peroxide
  - [ ] bandages
  - [ ] tweezers
  - [ ] over-the-counter pain medication
  - [ ] first aid booklet or pamphlet
- [ ] Hand sanitizer and moist towelettes
- [ ] Toilet paper or tissues

☐ Lighter and matches in waterproof container

☐ Heat pouches for body or hands

☐ Emergency blanket

☐ Windup or battery-powered flashlight
(and extra batteries)

☐ Windup or battery-operated radio (and extra batteries)

☐ Work gloves

☐ Whistle

☐ Pen/pencil and paper

☐ Small clock or watch

☐ Books, cards, games

☐ Photographs of family and pets

OTHER ITEMS _____

_____

_____

_____

_____

_____

_____

_____

Week 4 Checklist

☐ Review the Car Emergency Kit Supplies list to determine which items you already have.

☐ Shop for any items needed and assemble your car kit.

☐ Review the Emergency Work Kit Supplies list to determine which items you already have.

☐ Shop for any items needed and assemble your work kit.

☐ Review the Pet Emergency Kit Supplies list to determine which items you already have.

☐ Make copies of each pet's vaccination records to include in pet kit.

☐ Shop for any items needed and assemble your pet kit.

☐ List any tasks you need to complete or supplies you need to buy to finish the following:

    ☐ emergency communication plan

    ☐ home emergency kit

    ☐ home hazard elimination

    ☐ personal grab-and-go bag

    ☐ car emergency kit

    ☐ work emergency kit

    ☐ pet emergency kit

☐ Confirm the dates you have set to review your plans and refresh your supplies.

OTHER TASKS _____

Car Emergency Kit Supplies

☐ Copies of important documents, including:

    ☐ contact card (information about non-local emergency contacts completed in week 1)

    ☐ list of phone numbers

    ☐ car insurance

☐ Map of the area you live in

☐ Blanket

☐ Booster cables

☐ Fire extinguisher

☐ Spare car keys

☐ Cash—small-denomination bills and coins

☐ Water—at least 4 litres (1 gallon)

☐ Nonperishable snack such as granola bars or dried fruit

☐ Small first aid kit, including:

    ☐ hydrogen peroxide

    ☐ bandages

    ☐ tweezers

    ☐ over-the-counter pain medication

    ☐ first aid booklet or pamphlet

☐ Hand sanitizer and moist towelettes

☐ Toilet paper or tissues

☐ Lighter and matches in waterproof container

☐ Candles

- [ ] Windup or battery-powered flashlight (and extra batteries)
- [ ] Windup or battery-powered radio (and extra batteries)
- [ ] Work gloves
- [ ] Whistle
- [ ] Heavy-duty garbage bags
- [ ] Duct tape
- [ ] Pen/pencil and paper
- [ ] Book, cards, games
- [ ] Activity or colouring book and small stuffed animal for child

OTHER ITEMS _____

_____

_____

_____

_____

_____

_____

Work Emergency Kit Supplies

- ☐ Copies of important documents, including:
  - ☐ contact card (information about non-local emergency contacts completed in week 1)
  - ☐ list of phone numbers
  - ☐ Water—a least 1 litre (1 quart)
- ☐ Nonperishable snack such as granola bars or dried fruit
- ☐ Flat, comfortable walking shoes
- ☐ Socks
- ☐ Sweater
- ☐ Rain poncho or umbrella
- ☐ Small first aid kit, including:
  - ☐ hydrogen peroxide
  - ☐ bandages
  - ☐ tweezers
  - ☐ over-the-counter pain medication
  - ☐ first aid booklet or pamphlet
- ☐ Lighter and matches in waterproof container
- ☐ Candles
- ☐ Windup or battery-powered flashlight (and extra batteries)
- ☐ Windup or battery-powered radio (and extra batteries)
- ☐ Work gloves
- ☐ Whistle

OTHER ITEMS _____

Pet Emergency Kit Supplies

- ☐ Copies of vaccination records

- ☐ Spare leash and collar with ID tags

- ☐ Portable pet carrier

- ☐ Blanket or towel

- ☐ Dry or canned pet food
  (dry food is lightest and keeps longest)

- ☐ Can opener and a plastic lid for opening
  and storing canned food

- ☐ Water—at least 1 litre (1 quart)

- ☐ Bowls for water and food

- ☐ Prescription medication (enough for one week)

- ☐ Pet first aid kit, including:
  - ☐ hydrogen peroxide
  - ☐ bandages
  - ☐ gauze pads
  - ☐ cotton swabs
  - ☐ tweezers
  - ☐ appropriate pain medication
    (do not give aspirin to cats)
  - ☐ pet first aid booklet or pamphlet

- ☐ Sanitation supplies—plastic bags, paper towels,
  disposable wipes, kitty litter

- ☐ Brush or comb

- ☐ Toys and treats

OTHER ITEMS _____

What to Do When the Ground Shakes

DO NOT RUN OUTSIDE.

TAKE SHELTER.

- If you are inside, move under a sturdy table or desk.
- If no shelter inside is available, get down near an interior wall.
- If you are outside away from any buildings, trees, and power lines, stay put.
- If you are outside near tall buildings, move into a nearby doorway overhang or lobby.
- If you are outside on the street or sidewalk, move away from streetlights and utility poles.

DROP, COVER, AND HOLD ON.

- Drop down on to your hands and knees.
- Cover your head and neck.
- Hold on to your shelter.

DO NOT MOVE UNTIL THE SHAKING STOPS.

Fire Extinguisher Instructions

Place near extinguisher or attach to canister.

INSTRUCTIONS

> **P**ull the pin found at the top of the extinguisher to release the locking mechanism.

> **A**im the nozzle at the base of the fire to target the fuel that feeds the fire.

> **S**queeze the trigger slowly while holding the extinguisher upright.

> **S**weep from side to side covering the area of the fire.

RESOURCES

A MASSIVE amount of information on earthquakes and emergency preparedness is available on the Internet. The most reliable sources are sponsored by governments and associated organizations, or those affiliated with universities.

U.S. Geological Survey (USGS)

The Earthquake Hazards Program of the USGS (http://earthquake.usgs.gov) is the leading authority for current and historical global seismic information. As well as general earthquake information, the USGS has a reporting form and a wealth of fascinating maps:

> **Did You Feel It? form.** When you experience an earthquake you can submit a report about the shaking and damage. The USGS uses the data collected for research purposes and to develop maps.

> **Earthquake maps.** These are real-time, global maps that report earthquakes as they happen around the world. You can click on the epicentres of particular earthquake events and find out details such as location and magnitude.

> **ShakeMaps.** Within ten minutes of a seismic event (magnitude 3.5 or greater) the USGS displays a map showing the ground motion and intensity of shaking for the affected

area. The maps become increasingly more accurate over the days following an event as seismologists process the initial data and add incoming reports from local geology sources. These maps are used by government agencies for preparedness exercises and disaster planning and in larger earthquakes for real-time earthquake response and recovery.

> **Regional Maps.** High-risk regions have hazard maps. For example, detailed maps of potential earthquake hazards are provided for Seattle, Washington.

Earthquakes Canada
National Resources Canada (www.earthquakescanada. nrcan.gc.ca) provides information about earthquake detection and measurement in Canada. You can view the locations of seismographs and seismometers, see up-to-the-minute readings of seismic events, and find information about earthquake activity around the world.

Public Safety and Emergency Preparedness Canada
The 72 Hours campaign (www.GetPrepared.ca) encourages Canadians to be prepared to cope on their own for at least the first seventy-two hours of an emergency so that first responders can focus on those in urgent need. The campaign website provides information on assessing disaster risk and a downloadable emergency preparedness guide.

Other Organizations
- Federal Emergency Management Agency
  www.fema.gov

- Incorporated Research Institutions for Seismology
  www.iris.washington.edu

- International Tsunami Information Center
  http://itic.ioc-unesco.org

- National Oceanic and Atmospheric Administration
  http://tsunami.noaa.gov/prepare.html

- Provincial Emergency Program for British Columbia
  www.pep.bc.ca/hazard_preparedness/Earthquake_
  Information.html

- Pacific Disaster Center
  www.pdc.org/iweb/pdchome.htm

- Pacific Northwest Seismograph Network
  www.geophys.washington.edu

- Pacific Tsunami Warning Center
  www.prh.noaa.gov/ptwc

- Ready America
  www.ready.gov/america/index.html

- Seismological Society of America
  www.seismosoc.org

- Washington Emergency Management Division
  www.emd.wa.gov

REFERENCES

American Red Cross. "Web Users Increasingly Rely on Social
Media to Seek Help in a Disaster." http://rdcrss.org/crvkrR.

Bonanno, George A. "Loss, Trauma, and Human Resilience:
Have We Underestimated the Human Capacity to Thrive After
Extremely Aversive Events?" *American Psychologist* 59:1
(2004): 20–28.

Bond, Michael. "What Would You Do?" *Engineering and
Technology Magazine* 4:7 (2009). http://eandt.theiet.org/
magazine/2009/07/what-would-you-do.cfm.

Clague, John, Chris Yorath, and Richard Franklin. *At Risk:
Earthquakes and Tsunamis on the West Coast.* Vancouver:
Tricouni Press, 2006.

Cohen, Stanley. *States of Denial: Knowing about Atrocities
and Suffering.* Cambridge, UK: Polity, 2001.

Federal Emergency Management Agency (FEMA). Earthquake
Publications and Tools. www.fema.gov/plan/prevent/
earthquake/homeowners.shtm.

FEMA for Kids. "Earthquake Preparedness: What Every Childcare
Provider Should Know." Washington, DC: Federal Emergency
Management Agency, 1993. www.fema.gov/kids/tch_eq.htm.

Geological Survey of Canada. "Geodynamics—Cascadia
Subduction Zone." http://gsc.nrcan.gc.ca/geodyn/
cascadia_e.php.

Glass, T. "Understanding Public Response to Disasters."
  Public Health Reports 116 (2001): 69–73.

Humboldt State University. "Living on Shaky Ground—How to
  Survive Earthquakes and Tsunamis in Northern California."
  www.humboldt.edu/shakyground.

Laur, Darren. "The Anatomy of Fear and How It Relates to Survival
  Skills Training." Victoria: Integrated Street Combatives, 2002.
  www.lwcbooks.com/articles/anatomy.html.

Layton, Peggy Dianne. *Emergency Food Storage and Survival
  Handbook: Everything You Need to Know to Keep Your
  Family Safe in a Crisis.* New York: Three Rivers, 2004.

LeDoux, Joseph E. *The Emotional Brain: the Mysterious
  Underpinnings of Emotional Life.* New York: Simon &
  Schuster, 1996.

Marano, Lou. "Altruism, Not Panic, Prevails in Disasters."
  UPI.com. www.upi.com/view.cfm?StoryID=
  20020823-045931-6068r.

Mayse, Susan. *Earthquake: Surviving the Big One.* Auburn,
  WA: Lone Pine, 1992.

National Center for Disaster Preparedness. "The 2008 American
  Preparedness Project: Why Parents May Not Heed Evacuation
  Orders and What Emergency Planners, Families and Schools
  Need to Know." www.ncdp.mailman.columbia.edu/
  program_school.htm.

Provincial Emergency Program. "British Columbia Earthquake
  Response Plan (2008)." Victoria, BC: PEP, 2008.
  www.pep.bc.ca/hazard_plans/EQ_Plan.pdf.

Ripley, Amanda. "Why We Don't Prepare for Disaster."
  Time Magazine (August 20, 2006). www.time.com/time/
  magazine/article/0,9171,1229102,00.html.

Ripley, Amanda. *The Unthinkable: Who Survives When Disaster
  Strikes—and Why.* New York: Three Rivers, 2009.

Ropeik, David, and George Gray. *Risk: A Practical Guide for Deciding What's Really Safe and What's Dangerous in the World around You.* Boston: Houghton Mifflin, 2002.

Slovic, Paul. *The Perception of Risk.* London: Earthscan Publications, 2000.

Solnit, Rebecca. *A Paradise Built in Hell: The Extraordinary Communities That Arise in Disasters.* New York: Viking, 2009.

Spittal, Matthew, John McClure, Richard Siegert, and Frank Walkey. "Predictors of Two Types of Earthquake Preparation: Survival Activities and Mitigation." *Environment and Behavior* 40:6 (2008): 798–817.

Ulin, David L. *The Myth of Solid Ground: Earthquakes, Prediction, and the Fault Line between Reason and Faith.* New York: Viking, 2004.

U.S. Geological Survey. "What Are Aftershocks, Foreshocks and Earthquake Clusters?" http://earthquake.usgs.gov/earthquakes/step/explain.php.

Ventura, Michael. "The Earthquake People." *Psychology Today* (May 1, 1994). www.psychologytoday.com/articles/199405/the-earthquake-people.

Weinstein, Neil D. "Unrealistic Optimism about Susceptibility to Health Problems." *Journal of Behavioral Medicine* 5:4 (1982): 441–460.

Yanev, Peter I., and Andrew C.T. Thompson. *Peace of Mind in Earthquake Country: How to Save Your Home, Business, and Life.* San Francisco: Chronicle, 2008.

Yeats, Robert S. *Living with Earthquakes in the Pacific Northwest.* Corvallis: Oregon State University Press, 2004.

INDEX

MAGGIE MOONEY is a writer and a community facilitator with a master's degree in counselling psychology. She is author of *Canada's Top 100: The Greatest Athletes of All Time* and co-author of *Nobel's Women of Peace*. She lives on Gabriola Island in the Cascadia subduction zone.

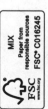